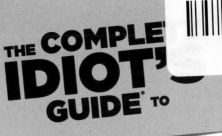

The Coconut Oil Diet

by Maria Blanco, CFH, and Dr. James Pendleton, ND, NMD

ALPHA

A member of Penguin Group (USA) Inc.

ALPHA BOOKS

Published by Penguin Group (USA) Inc.

Penguin Group (USA) Inc., 375 Hudson Street, New York, New York 10014, USA • Penguin Group (Canada), 90 Eglinton Avenue East, Suite 700, Toronto, Ontario M4P 2Y3, Canada (a division of Pearson Penguin Canada Inc.) • Penguin Books Ltd., 80 Strand, London WC2R 0RL, England • Penguin Ireland, 25 St. Stephen's Green, Dublin 2, Ireland (a division of Penguin Books Ltd.) • Penguin Group (Australia), 250 Camberwell Road, Camberwell, Victoria 3124, Australia (a division of Pearson Australia Group Pty. Ltd.) • Penguin Books India Pvt. Ltd., 11 Community Centre, Panchsheel Park, New Delhi—110 017, India • Penguin Group (NZ), 67 Apollo Drive, Rosedale, North Shore, Auckland 1311, New Zealand (a division of Pearson New Zealand Ltd.) • Penguin Books (South Africa) (Pty.) Ltd., 24 Sturdee Avenue, Rosebank, Johannesburg 2196, South Africa • Penguin Books Ltd., Registered Offices: 80 Strand, London WC2R 0RL, England

International Standard Book Number: 978-1-61564-257-1
Library of Congress Catalog Card Number: 2012951732

15 14 13   8 7 6 5 4 3 2 1

Interpretation of the printing code: The rightmost number of the first series of numbers is the year of the book's printing; the rightmost number of the second series of numbers is the number of the book's printing. For example, a printing code of 13-1 shows that the first printing occurred in 2013.

Printed in the United States of America

Note: This publication contains the opinions and ideas of its authors. It is intended to provide helpful and informative material on the subject matter covered. It is sold with the understanding that the authors and publisher are not engaged in rendering professional services in the book. If the reader requires personal assistance or advice, a competent professional should be consulted.

The authors and publisher specifically disclaim any responsibility for any liability, loss, or risk, personal or otherwise, which is incurred as a consequence, directly or indirectly, of the use and application of any of the contents of this book.

Most Alpha books are available at special quantity discounts for bulk purchases for sales promotions, premiums, fund-raising, or educational use. Special books, or book excerpts, can also be created to fit specific needs. For details, write: Special Markets, Alpha Books, 375 Hudson Street, New York, NY 10014.

Publisher: *Mike Sanders*
Executive Managing Editor: *Billy Fields*
Acquisitions Editor: *Tom Stevens*
Senior Development Editor: *Christy Wagner*
Development Editor: *Nancy Lewis*
Senior Production Editor: *Kayla Dugger*

Copy Editor: *Amy Lepore*
Cover Designer: *Rebecca Batchelor*
Book Designers: *William Thomas, Rebecca Batchelor*
Indexer: *Julie Bess*
Layout: *Ayanna Lacey*
Proofreader: *Virginia Vought*

Contents

Introduction

If improving your health in the most natural way possible is important to you, then this book will provide you with a treasure trove of information. The health benefits of including coconut oil in your diet and in routine self-care are phenomenal and far-reaching. In this book you will discover wonderful things about coconut oil and about health in general that you have never heard. Best of all, I've broken all this exciting information down into easy-to-understand chunks so that you can dive right in anywhere and get started right away.

The coconut oil diet focuses on consuming the healthy fats and foods that our ancestors thrived on from time immemorial. It teaches you how to eat healthily for a lifetime and how to naturally avoid and overcome illness and disease. In the recipes in the last part of the book, you will discover the basis of real nutrition. You'll have more energy. You'll lose those nagging cravings. Your weight will finally normalize. You will achieve a level of wellness you maybe never thought possible. And you'll be astonished to witness how fast your cholesterol and blood pressure go down, even as your energy levels soar.

How This Book Is Organized

I've broken this book into four parts to make it easier for you to find the information you need to personally tailor a coconut oil diet plan that's right for you. Each part provides foundational information, hints and tips on which to build.

Part 1, Coconut Oil Basics, explores the marvelous health claims surrounding coconut oil and provides quizzes that help you determine how coconut oil can be of benefit to you. You will learn about coconut oil's interesting historical legacy. You'll also discover that coconut oil was once considered a highly valuable dietary fat and how, in recent times, events conspired to give coconut oil an undeserved bad reputation. Finally, you will learn that coconut oil is available in a variety of forms and an exciting array of world-class cuisines.

Part 2, The Science Behind Coconut Oil, dives directly into the business of how and why coconut oil is able to accomplish so many amazing feats. It discusses the medium-chain fatty acids in coconut oil and their long list of health-promoting attributes. Fascinating scientific studies conducted on coconut oil and among the societies who have used it most are also explored. The end of Part 2 navigates you through comparisons of coconut oil to other fats and explains why coconut oil possesses superior benefits in the diet with none of the drawbacks of modern vegetable oils.

Part 3, The Myriad Health Benefits of Coconut Oil, digs deep to uncover all the ways coconut oil is useful as a nutraceutical ally—a food that can provide health benefits, including the prevention and treatment of disease. Coconut oil's ability to conquer the HIV virus, reverse symptoms of Alzheimer's disease, contribute to heart health, enhance and improve thyroid function, help you achieve a healthy weight, and produce healthy skin and hair are all covered in Part 3. Helpful tips on how to use coconut oil for each condition are included, along with explanations of how coconut oil gets the job done.

Part 4, Coconut Oil Recipes, is where the rubber meets the road. You will discover wonderful recipes to put all of your newly acquired coconut oil knowledge into practice. Chapter 15 introduces exotic recipes that explore coconut cuisine from the tropical shores of Tahiti, India, Hawaii, and Samoa. Next you'll delve into the incredible versatility of coconut in Chapter 16's exciting soups, curries, and condiments, featuring recipes from Thailand and Brazil. Chapter 17 is where the sweets and treats are found. It also provides delightful coconut recipes that fit the high standards of dementia patients and acknowledges the time constraints of caregivers' needs. The final chapter provides recipes of a different kind. Because coconut oil nourishes the body from the outside, too, this chapter offers recipes for natural homemade hygiene, hair, and skin-care products.

The appendixes are an added bonus for you. You'll find sources for coconut oil edibles and skin-care products, hard-to-find nutrition supplements, and exotic foods in Appendix A. There is also a "Further Reading" list in Appendix B that introduces you to wonderful print and online resources to explore.

Extras

Throughout the book, I've included sidebars that point out tips, cautions, definitions, and extra information about the coconut oil diet. Here's what to look for:

DEFINITION

These sidebars provide you with the meaning of terms that are relevant to the topic at hand.

AW, NUTS!

These sidebars provide you with warnings about matters that can affect your health or seriously compromise expected results.

TO YOUR HEALTH!

These sidebars provide interesting and helpful background information on coconut oil, research, and expert opinions.

TROPICAL TIP

These sidebars provide hints for making the use of coconut oil easier or give advice that increases your understanding.

But Wait! There's More!

Have you logged on to idiotsguides.com lately? If you haven't, go there now! As a bonus to the book, we've included tons of additional information, such as at-home spa treatments using coconut oil, how to make your own virgin coconut oil at home, and several sweets and dessert recipes made with coconut flour. You'll want to check them out, all online. Point your browser to idiotsguides.com/coconutoildiet, and enjoy!

Acknowledgments

On a very personal level, I would like to thank the late Dr. J. Alvin Mayer for having been my mentor and physician in the great tradition of the Latin *docere* (doctor as teacher). In caring for your patients, you were brave and fearless in your convictions and considered opinions despite any resultant consternation or inconvenience. Your inspired curiosity and enthusiasm to broach any medical subject—even with a child, and regardless of the time it might have required—will ever endear you to me.

I would also like to acknowledge the monumental contributions made in the fields of science, nutrition and medicine by: Weston A. Price, DDS; Francis M. Pottenger, MD; William H. Philpott, MD; Linus Pauling, PhD; Robert C. Atkins, MD; Mary G. Enig, PhD; Michael Holick, PhD, MD; and Howard F. Loomis, DC.

For their insights, expertise, and great generosity, special thanks also go to Brian and Marianita Shilhavy of Tropical Traditions, Robert Schueller of Melissa's Produce, and the Weston A. Price Foundation.

Tremendous gratitude is due my loving supportive parents, Roland and Laura Hebert, for the legacy of my Cajun heritage which honors the inherent wisdom of traditional nutrition and culture; and to my father especially, who enthusiastically explored and reproduced the finest of traditional world cuisines, with and for me, throughout our travels. *Equal* love and gratitude to my Cotton family, to whom I owe my very life and so much more.

Finally and foremost, a deep, heartfelt *thank you* to my husband Dewayne and to our children who have unwaveringly supported me through my writing endeavors, and who have been tireless cheerleaders for "the cause" that they may not have always understood. *Ad Majorem Dei Gloriam, Anno Domini MMXII.*

Special Thanks to My Team

Very special thanks go to Marilyn Allen of Allen O'Shea Literary Agency and to Lori Hand, my acquisitions editor at Alpha Books, for having such enthusiastic faith and confidence in me, and for their warm support and expert guidance throughout this exciting project.

To my friend, Dr. James Pendleton: Many heartfelt thanks for reviewing this book for accuracy and for offering the benefit of your talents as both writer and physician.

Trademarks

Coconut Oil Basics

Every week there is a new take in the news about what foods are healthy (and not so healthy) to consume. On any given day, the same food that one article proclaims to be a new miracle food is simultaneously lambasted in another article as having been associated with some terrible disease. One of the latest media buzzes is all about the health benefits of coconut oil. What's a person to believe?

Part 1 explores the validity of the health claims surrounding coconut oil. It covers common disorders that coconut oil is claimed to relieve and provides quizzes to help you determine whether you might benefit from adding coconut oil to your diet. Next we transition to coconut oil's historical use and the excellent health that coconut-dependent cultures have traditionally enjoyed. In addition, we explain how coconut oil once was a highly valued and important dietary oil throughout the world—and how it eventually came to have an undeserved bad reputation. Finally, you will discover the many ways of sourcing coconut oil for your own diet and be introduced to the concept of the coconut oil diet itself.

Coconut Oil: What's All the Buzz About?

In This Chapter

- Following coconut oil in the news
- Understanding how coconut oil supports health
- Quizzing yourself for potential improved health
- Realizing the truth behind panaceas

If you follow current health news and dietary recommendations, you have no doubt heard something about coconut oil. Lately, the health buzz surrounding coconut oil has reached a level of near frenzy.

While older studies have reported that coconut oil is a killer fat and should be avoided like the plague, there are newer reports to the contrary. These exciting articles state that coconut oil is not only good for you, but can treat and cure all sorts of diseases.

Of course, when there is so much hype about something, it's prudent to find out how much truth is contained in all those glowing reports. Well, in the case of virgin coconut oil, it turns out that most of the "hype" is amazingly true.

The Easiest Path to Improved Health

When educating clients about healthy food choices, I find that many of them are surprised and dismayed to hear that coconut oil is at the top of my "Top 10" healthiest foods list because they have heard that tropical oils are made up of saturated fats that should be avoided.

Coconut oil ranks so high because of its nutritional value, but also because of its potential for promoting healing and its ability to aid in disease prevention.

Maybe you are reading this book because you want to lose a few pounds, or maybe you want to say good-bye to some nagging health issues. Well, I have good news for you. The fastest and easiest way to achieve your goal is to systematically add high-quality foods to your diet. Eventually, you will have added so many good things that the bad stuff will be edged out. So let's get started on your journey to a new, healthier you by adding coconut oil to your diet—today.

TO YOUR HEALTH!

Studies from the 1960s and 1970s show that Asians and Pacific Islanders whose diets were rich in coconut oil were substantially free of cardiovascular disease despite consuming 35 to 60 percent of their calories in the form of saturated fat. While the consumption of saturated fat has long been considered a main contributing factor to the development of cardiovascular disease in the West, the findings of these studies directly contradict many traditional doctors' recommendations to limit them.

Coconut Oil as Medicine

The coconut is a nutritious source of nutmeat, water, milk, and oil that has sustained many populations around the world for untold generations. Coconut is a staple in the diet of many tropical cultures, and it is often the major component of every meal. In fact, nearly 30 percent of the world's population is in some way dependent on coconut for survival. Among these people, coconut enjoys a longstanding, highly revered reputation.

Yet modern science has only recently begun to understand what traditional island cultures have always known. Coconut is not only highly nutritious; it provides health benefits that greatly surpass what can be explained by its nutritional profile alone. In nutrition circles, such foods are known as "functional foods." Other examples of functional foods are: oats, for their fiber content which has been shown to lower cholesterol; tomatoes, whose lycopene content reduces cancer risk; and garlic, which when crushed develops sulfur compounds containing cancer-preventative, antibiotic, antihypertensive, and cholesterol-lowering properties.

Pacific Islanders recognize this functionality and consider the coconut's oil, in particular, to be a cure for all illness. In the islands, the precious palm that bears the coconut "medicine" is known as the "Tree of Life." To call coconut oil a medicine, however, might be a mistake—at least as far as the U.S. Food and Drug Administration (FDA) is concerned. Regardless, it is certainly a healthy and beneficial food—one of the healthiest foods on Earth.

TO YOUR HEALTH!

In a 1986 court case, a firm that marketed and distributed blue-green algae (an all-natural food) insisted that its products were food supplements and therefore did not require FDA approval. It also claimed, however, that the supplements would improve mental clarity and memory; increase energy and vitality; improve sleep; relieve fatigue, hypoglycemia, some allergies, and poor digestion; promote weight loss and detoxification; and provide an overall increased sense of well-being and stamina.

The FDA contended, however, that by claiming the food could alleviate symptoms of several maladies, the firm had inadvertently "created" a new drug. The judge agreed with the FDA's position, which was that the food product should not be allowed on the market.

The moral of the story: although it is a widely accepted fact that a few particular foods can help to prevent and correct certain diseases, saying so might be against the law.

The Secret Ingredient for Vibrant Health

In 1981, the *American Journal of Clinical Nutrition* published studies by Dr. Ian Prior and Flora Davidson that were conducted among the South Pacific's Pukapuka and Tokelau Islanders. Despite the islanders' high consumption of saturated fat in the form of coconut oil and lard, health problems such as atherosclerosis, heart disease, colon cancer, kidney disease, and high serum cholesterol were virtually unknown. The people were found to be lean and healthy.

The uniquely structured molecules of the saturated fatty acids in coconut oil appear to be the key. Coconut oil is mostly composed of *medium-chain triglycerides* (*MCTs*)—lauric, capric, and caprylic acids in particular.

- Lauric acid is a major and vital component of mothers' milk and plays an important role in an infant's growth, development, and immunity.
- Capric acid and caprylic acid both fight yeast and fungal overgrowth.

These MCTs have been found to dissolve gallstones, destroy the HIV virus, and enhance the production of insulin by the pancreas. MCTs are also very stable at high temperatures, which can prevent rancidity and tissue-damaging free radical formation (see Chapter 7).

If this were not enough, the fatty acids in coconut oil work to kill lipid-encapsulated viruses and bacteria, too, including many sexually transmitted diseases such as chlamydia and AIDS (see Chapter 8).

Therapeutically, MCTs have shown value in the treatment of *cachexia*, dementia, and childhood epilepsy. The MCTs in coconut oil have proven helpful in preventing or relieving all of these conditions and many more.

DEFINITION

Medium-chain triglycerides (MCTs) are 6- to 12-carbon medium-chain fatty acids. MCTs passively move from the GI tract to the portal vein system without needing modification before they can be assimilated, unlike long-chain fatty acids (more than 12 carbons) or very-long-chain fatty acids (more than 22 carbons). MCTs are immediately available and go to work fulfilling cells' energy requirements.

Cachexia is a syndrome of progressive weight loss, anorexia, and loss of muscle and body mass. It is often seen in cancer patients as a response to a malignant growth.

Can Coconut Oil Help Me, Too?

Coconut oil has such a long list of health benefits that the simple answer is probably *yes*. But to get a clearer idea of how adding

coconut oil to your diet may improve your health, take a look at the
following health quizzes.

Thyroid Health Quiz

Hypothyroidism is one of the most underdiagnosed hormonal
disorders in America. The thyroid gland controls metabolism, body
temperature, and the production of stomach acid and digestive
enzymes. It regulates how your body uses food energy, burns fat, and
synthesizes protein. It even plays a vital role in the regulation and
synthesis of sex hormones.

Check each box that applies:

- ❑ My basal body temperature before arising is below 97.4°F.
- ❑ I feel weak or lethargic.
- ❑ I'm sluggish and achy in the morning.
- ❑ My face and/or eyelids are puffy.
- ❑ My skin, hair, and nails are dry, coarse, or brittle.
- ❑ I've gained weight and can't seem to get it back to normal.
- ❑ I feel depressed.
- ❑ The outer edges of my eyebrows are disappearing.
- ❑ I have PMS or irregular, long, or heavy menstruation.
- ❑ My scalp or body hair is thinning.
- ❑ I'm easily or chronically constipated.
- ❑ I'm sensitive to cold.
- ❑ I have infertility problems.
- ❑ I experience "brain fog" or short-term memory loss.
- ❑ My pulse rate is too slow or too rapid.
- ❑ I have high or low blood pressure.
- ❑ I have high cholesterol.
- ❑ My voice has become huskier, deeper, or hoarse sounding.
- ❑ I've had one or more miscarriages.
- ❑ I've had postpartum depression and/or difficulty nursing.
- ❑ I have low libido (sex drive).
- ❑ My eyes are red, inflamed, gritty feeling, or bulging.

❑ I experience blurry or double vision.

❑ I have bothersome allergies.

❑ I have sleep apnea.

❑ I experience vertigo (dizziness with the illusion of motion) and/or tinnitus (ringing in the ears).

❑ I sense a fullness/discomfort in my neck.

❑ Neckties and turtlenecks are very uncomfortable.

If you checked seven or more boxes, you probably should have your thyroid function evaluated. Ask your doctor for a test that shows levels of TSH, free T3 and T4, along with the "normal ranges" for each value.

TO YOUR HEALTH!

Removing goitrogens (substances that interfere with thyroid function, like soy and soy by-products) from your diet and replacing polyunsaturated vegetable oils with virgin coconut oil can help to support healthy thyroid function.

Yeast and Fungal Overgrowth Quiz

Yeast and fungal overgrowth have become a plague to modern society, mostly due to the overconsumption of sugary and starchy foods in the Western diet and the rampant use of antibiotics that kill off competing protective bacteria.

Yeast and fungi often infect mucus membranes such as those found in the vagina, mouth, and sinuses. They also grow happily in moist areas of the skin such as between toes and in the groin area, navel, and skin folds. But left unchecked, yeast can overgrow and infect any organ of the body and do considerable damage in the process. Some common names for these and related conditions include candidiasis, thrush, sprue, ringworm, and jock itch.

Check each box that applies:

❑ I take antibiotics frequently.

❑ I have taken 10 or more courses of antibiotics (oral or IV) in my lifetime.

❑ I have routinely taken tetracycline for acne.

❑ I have experienced recurrent vaginitis or persistent prostatitis.

❑ I experience itching of the vagina, penis, groin, and/or rectum.

❑ I have a vaginal discharge (white, off-white, or cottage cheese–like).

❑ I am now or have been pregnant.

❑ I have had multiple pregnancies.

❑ I have taken birth control pills.

❑ I have been on birth control (subdermal implants, IUDs, diaphragms, or spermicides) for more than two years.

❑ I have taken prednisone or corticosteroids.

❑ I have been diagnosed with ulcerative colitis, gluten intolerance, or Crohn's disease.

❑ I have a reaction to perfumes, new fabric odors, aerosols, and other chemical odors.

❑ I feel worse on damp, humid days.

❑ I have had ringworm, jock itch, or fungal infections of my nails or nail beds.

❑ I crave sugar, breads, or alcohol.

❑ I have a reaction to tobacco smoke.

❑ I have itchy skin or scalp.

❑ I have a low white blood cell (WBC) count.

❑ I have a feeling of being in a mental fog, spacey, or surreal.

❑ I have abdominal pain, constipation, or endometriosis.

Only a clinical evaluation by your physician can positively diagnose candidiasis, so if you have checked seven or more boxes, you may want to explore the matter further with your doctor.

TO YOUR HEALTH!

Topically applied coconut oil and a healthy, low-carbohydrate diet that includes coconut oil can help to kill off overgrowths of candida yeast and tinea fungal infections.

Fibromyalgia/Chronic Fatigue Syndrome Quiz

Many health professionals believe that the underlying cause of fibromyalgia and chronic fatigue syndrome is a depressed immune system, aggravated by hypothyroidism or by the Epstein-Barr or herpes virus. The core feature of these chronic disorders is pain, but other symptoms abound.

Check each box that applies:

- ❏ I have chronic muscle pain, spasms, or tightness.
- ❏ My pain has lasted more than three months.
- ❏ My pain is widespread—above and below my waist.
- ❏ I am fatigued and have low energy.
- ❏ I wake up feeling tired or have insomnia.
- ❏ I have stiffness and pain upon waking.
- ❏ I have stiffness and pain if I stay in one position too long.
- ❏ I have abdominal pain, bloating, or nausea.
- ❏ I have bouts of alternating constipation and diarrhea.
- ❏ I experience trouble concentrating.
- ❏ I experience tension headaches or migraines.
- ❏ My jaw and face are tender.
- ❏ I'm sensitive to odors, noises, bright lights, certain foods/ medicines, and cold.
- ❏ I have anxiety and/or depression.
- ❏ I have tingling or numbness in my face, hands, feet, arms, or legs.
- ❏ My urinary urgency/frequency has increased.
- ❏ Simple things that don't hurt others (like a hug) cause me real pain.

If you experience marked chronic pain and have checked seven or more boxes, you have a substantial number of fibromyalgia symptoms and may benefit from adding coconut oil to your diet.

The special fatty acids in coconut oil have the ability to kill giardia protozoa and certain viruses like herpes and Epstein-Barr—thereby reducing your viral load and allowing your immune system to function more efficiently. Many fibromyalgia sufferers report reduced pain and a return to normal living after adding coconut oil to their diets.

Hydrogenated Fats Quiz

Numerous studies have found that trans-fats raise our risk of heart disease. They also contribute to an increase in total serum cholesterol and a drop in healthy HDL cholesterol. These manufactured fats are toxic and have been associated with cancer and a long list of chronic disease conditions.

Check each of the listed foods you eat at least once per month:

- ❑ Margarine
- ❑ Commercial peanut butter
- ❑ Nondairy creamer
- ❑ Imitation whipping cream
- ❑ Microwaveable popcorn
- ❑ Commercial crackers
- ❑ Commercial snack cakes, cookies, or doughnuts
- ❑ Restaurant or frozen pizza
- ❑ Breaded fish or meats
- ❑ Cheese puffs, corn chips, or potato chips
- ❑ Frozen french fries, tater tots, or hash browns
- ❑ Tacos, tortillas, or burritos
- ❑ Boxed meals and meal "helpers"
- ❑ Commercial cakes or boxed cake mix
- ❑ Instant refrigerator biscuits or rolls
- ❑ Hamburger or hot dog buns
- ❑ Processed canned, boxed, or sliced cheese
- ❑ Creamed soups or frozen creamed vegetables
- ❑ Toaster pastries, egg rolls, pot pies, or calzones
- ❑ Sandwich cookies or jelly candies
- ❑ Commercial cold breakfast cereals
- ❑ Boxed soup mixes or side dishes

❑ Artichoke hearts bottled or canned in oil

❑ Boxed gelatin or pudding desserts

If you checked 13 or more of these foods, you may be suffering from hydrogenated oil toxicity.

Signs of hydrogenated oil toxicity consist of the development of chronic debilitating disease states. There are no overt symptoms before major damage has been done. The consumption of hydrogenated oils or trans-fats has been associated with cardiovascular disease, dementias, Parkinson's disease, multiple sclerosis, cancer, lupus, and other autoimmune disorders. Eating homemade foods using virgin coconut oil and fresh ingredients instead of commercially processed trans-fatty foods will reduce your risk of developing these disorders (see Chapter 7).

Parasite Quiz

You may think that parasites are a thing of the past or something only seen in remote areas of third-world countries. Nothing could be further from the truth.

Parasite infestations are common and cause a great deal of suffering in modern times. In some cases, the infestation can become epidemic, as in the 1993 Milwaukee parasite crisis where some 400,000 people contracted cryptosporidium from the city's water supply. Cryptosporidium is a gastrointestinal protozoan parasite which causes watery diarrhea, dehydration, weight loss, stomach cramps, pain, fever, nausea, and vomiting. Half the city's population was affected and several people died.

Check each box that applies:

❑ I am a restless sleeper.

❑ I have persistent joint pain.

❑ I'm nearly always anemic.

❑ I sometimes forget to wash my hands before handling food or after using the restroom.

❑ I drink unfiltered water.

❑ I travel overseas and/or to Mexico.

❑ I live or have lived in the tropics.

❑ I lived overseas before moving to the United States.

❑ I own a cat or dog.

❑ I eat raw fish or meats.

❑ I eat homemade sausages.

❑ I like my steaks rare or "blue" (rarer than rare).

❑ I have rectal itching or pressure.

❑ I have muscle weakness and wasting.

❑ I'm always hungry.

❑ My skin itches and is worse at night.

❑ I have dark circles under my eyes.

❑ I can't seem to gain weight.

❑ I have unexplained weight loss.

❑ I have night sweats and/or insomnia.

❑ I have abdominal pain or bloating.

❑ My stools are poorly formed.

❑ I have mucus in my stools and/or diarrhea.

❑ I am almost always tired and fatigued.

❑ I've been diagnosed with ulcerative colitis.

❑ I've been diagnosed with Crohn's disease.

If you have checked seven or more boxes, you may want to have your doctor test you for an intestinal parasite infestation and modify your diet in ways that aid your body in its efforts to eliminate them.

Coconut oil contains a high percentage of lauric acid, which is converted by the body into monolaurin, a substance that efficiently kills many parasites, yeasts, viruses, and bacteria that reside in the gut.

Inappropriate Estrogen Quiz

If you are a woman, estrogen is a good thing—right? Well, it's not quite that simple. Levels of estrogen can be inappropriate in that sometimes levels can be too high and become toxic. Or they can be inappropriate in relationship to the levels of other hormones in the body.

Besides the estrogens that our own bodies create, we are constantly bombarded by environmental estrogens from plastics and by phytoestrogen sources in our foods—especially the ever-present soy oils and soy by-products. It has been proposed that these external sources of estrogen may be at the root of the very real increase in precocious (early-onset) puberty among girls, as well as an alleged increase in effeminate traits among developing boys.

Check each box that applies:

- ❑ I experience night sweats, hot flashes, or insomnia.
- ❑ I have low libido (sex drive).
- ❑ I suffer from PMS and heavy or painful periods.
- ❑ I have gynecomastia (enlarged breasts in men).
- ❑ I am obese or substantially overweight.
- ❑ I have a family history of reproductive cancer.
- ❑ I experience uncomfortable vaginal dryness.
- ❑ I am experiencing erectile dysfunction.
- ❑ I am experiencing infertility problems.
- ❑ I have a family history of ovarian cysts.
- ❑ My breasts become painful/swollen before or during my periods.
- ❑ Fibrocystic breast disease runs in my family.
- ❑ I suffer from endometriosis.
- ❑ I use birth control pills or implants.
- ❑ I have had abnormal PAP smear results.
- ❑ I have excessive facial hair (women).
- ❑ I follow a strictly low-fat diet.

If you are a woman who has marked seven or more of these boxes (or a man who has marked 5 or more), you may want to explore your hormone balance further with your doctor.

Ensure you are getting an abundance of fresh whole foods in your diet every day. Whole foods support your body's natural ability to balance hormones. Include brightly colored vegetables and fruits, as well as hormone-free sources of protein.

Avoid refined vegetable oils (such as soybean oil, canola oil, and corn oil) in your diet and substitute healthy fats like coconut oil, extra-virgin olive oil, fats from organic free-range dairy products, and fish oil. Also try to avoid exposure to plastics and highly estrogenic foods like soy products, as these can contribute to estrogen dominance.

Is Coconut Oil a Panacea?

The quizzes in the previous section may have convinced you that coconut oil is an important tool in the management of several common problems. But coconut oil's alleged health benefits number in the hundreds, perhaps even the thousands.

So it is understandable that the coconut palm or "Tree of Life" (as traditional cultures of the Pacific Islands refer to it) is believed to produce the "medicine that cures all ills." In fact, anyone looking for a *panacea* in the future should be sure to include coconut oil on the vetting list.

> **DEFINITION**
>
> **Panacea** was the goddess of healing in Greek mythology. The daughter of Aesculapius and the sister of Hygeia, Panacea was said to possess a poultice that could cure all disease. Perhaps inspired by the Greek myth, ancient alchemists searched in vain for a **panacea** (lowercase) that would remedy all sickness and disease.

As it turns out, herbs like heal-all (*Prunella vulgaris*), aspirin (salicylic acid) from white willow bark, and penicillin from blue-green bread mold have each been proclaimed, in turn, a panacea by well-meaning if overly optimistic enthusiasts.

The truth is, however, that medicines don't heal—none of them do. Foods don't heal and doctors can't heal either. It is the body that heals itself. Healing takes place in the body naturally, and it is exactly what the body always strives for when it is not well.

As long as the body receives sufficient quality nutrition, a safe and nontoxic environment, fresh air, and clean water, the body tends to heal. All the body's various systems naturally tend toward healing and balance through a process known as *homeostasis*. Once that balance has been established, health naturally prevails.

DEFINITION

Homeostasis is the tendency of the body's systems to remain stable while also adjusting to conditions that are optimal for survival. Homeostatic mechanisms are necessary for the body to maintain balance and to regain balance when dealing with disease or injury.

Coconut oil is a functional food that assists the body in its attempts at achieving and maintaining homeostasis. It provides the body with tools it can use in eliminating viral, bacterial, and fungal invaders, simultaneously providing unique, high-quality nourishment.

Because a panacea began as a mythical concept, perhaps that is also where the notion of a medicinal panacea should be left. There is no such thing as a panacea—neither in the realm of medicine, nor in that of food. But virgin coconut oil certainly comes close because it gives the body so much of what it needs in its amazing work of growing, building, cleansing, healing, and repairing.

The Least You Need to Know

- Coconut oil supports health by providing unique nutrition in the form of MCTs that are instantly available to cells for growth, maintenance, repair, and enhanced immune function.
- Ancient cultures knew coconut oil's health-giving properties and referred to it as the "Tree of Life."
- Medium-chain triglycerides in coconut oil—like lauric acid, capric acid, and caprylic acid—kill viruses, bacteria, and parasites.
- Replacing estrogenic soy oils and free-radical-producing refined vegetable oils with the stable saturated fatty acids found in coconut oil can help the body to naturally establish healthy hormonal balance.
- There are no panaceas, but coconut oil comes close.

Coconut Oil's Traditional Use and History

In This Chapter

* Learning the truth about coconut oil's history
* Did conspiracy kill the coconut oil industry?
* Choosing the best coconut oil

Traditional tropical cultures have historically enjoyed vibrant health, youthful skin, beautiful hair, and toned, trim bodies. It's part of the picture of paradise—isn't it? Everybody wants that.

There is reason to think that the secret to the vibrant health enjoyed by tropical cultures is the high content of coconut oil in their traditional diet.

But, you say, *aren't tropical oils bad for us?* It's true that tropical oils have received very bad press in recent years. But it was not always that way. This chapter explores how coconut oil came to have such a bad reputation and why it is completely unfounded. You'll also learn about the different types of coconut oil and why they are not all equal.

Tropical Origins

Traditionally, in health class we are told that to maintain health and to avoid obesity and chronic degenerative disease, we need to reduce calories and avoid saturated fats. Yet, in the tropics, it turns out that this rule holds no water. Tropical cultures, eating their customary high-fat, high-calorie diets—diets rich in saturated fats and cholesterol—have enjoyed examples of the most robust health.

> **TO YOUR HEALTH!**
>
> In the 1930s, Dr. Weston A. Price visited and conducted extensive studies among traditional cultures throughout the world, as documented in his book, *Nutrition and Physical Degeneration: A Comparison of Primitive and Modern Diets and Their Effects.*

The extensive research of Dr. Weston A. Price in the 1920s and 1930s, and that of Dr. Ian A. Prior published in 1981, bear this out. Price found that all diets were high in saturated plant and animal fats, which provided as much as 60 percent of their caloric intake. There were no vegetarians. The diet of these healthy indigenous peoples provided at least ten times the vitamin A and D of modern Western diets and at least four times the amount of other vitamins and minerals. Price's research concluded that various aspects of modern diets such as refined vegetable oils, flours, and sugars, result in nutritional deficiencies that are at the root of many modern health problems and debilitating diseases.

Dr. Prior conducted epidemiological research throughout the Pacific, most notably among the people of the Pukapuka and Tokelau Islands. His research included a broader spectrum of people than many researchers who had gone before him and included women. Prior's work identified a connection between heart disease and excessive salt intake and he outlined how modern diets are linked to chronic disease and obesity.

Price and Prior found that people of the tropics, who had not adopted modern ways of eating, did not suffer from heart disease, diabetes, or any of the typical chronic conditions so common in the developed world. Even today, in humid, tropical environments where there is such a great proliferation of fungi, yeast, and bacteria, native peoples who adhere to their dietary traditions do not get yeast and fungal infestations. Bacteria stay in check and don't cause overt infection, and among these people modern disease is still relatively rare. So it would behoove us to discover how traditional tropical cultures have lived and what they have held as valuable in their diets.

Coconut's Role in the Traditional Diet

Native wild coconut grows in a surprisingly broad swath of the globe: in more than 80 countries, mostly concentrated in the islands and along the shores of tropical and equatorial regions. Notable cultures include those of the Philippines, Indonesia, Brazil, Thailand, Polynesia, and India. In coastal India, the coconut palm is also called *Kalpavriksha*, the "tree that gives all that is necessary for living."

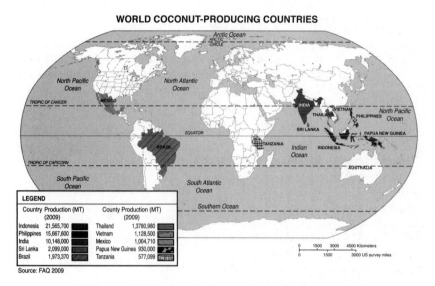

WORLD COCONUT-PRODUCING COUNTRIES

LEGEND			
Country Production (MT) (2009)		County Production (MT) (2009)	
Indonesia	21,565,700	Thailand	1,3780,980
Philippines	15,667,600	Vietnam	1,128,500
India	10,148,000	Mexico	1,004,710
Sri Lanka	2,099,000	Papua New Guinea	930,000
Brazil	1,973,370	Tanzania	577,099

Source: FAQ 2009

Coconut oil production throughout the equatorial and tropical regions of the globe.

Prior to the 1950s, most tropical cultures still lived in small rural communities and earned their livings from what nature provided. Today this would be termed an "organic existence." In areas such as the Philippine islands, people were primarily farmers and fishermen. Farmers planted, grew, and harvested by hand all of the crops their families needed—rice, vegetables and root crops like taro, and herbs like garlic and ginger. But their primary source of food and income was wild-growing coconut, for which there was a thriving world market—especially in the baking industry.

Coconut and coconut oil were used in the traditional diet every day. The coconut oil was processed at home, by hand, using a method that employed either natural fermentation or boiling. It was used in frying all types of foods and in the preparation of rice and vegetables.

Farmers fed coconut meat to livestock, including chickens and hogs. Even the poorest of families had coconut flesh and *buko juice* to give their children, and the people and their animals enjoyed vibrant health.

DEFINITION

Buko juice is the clear liquid (coconut water) inside young coconuts. It is a very popular drink in the tropics, especially in Southeast Asia, the Pacific Islands, Africa, and the Caribbean. Lately it has become available canned or bottled and is now being marketed as a natural sports drink due to its healthy high-mineral content.

Traditional Native Production

In traditional cultures, natural fermentation has been employed in processing and preserving foods. Examples of this include beverages such as wine, beer, and kvass; dairy items such as cheese, yogurt, and kefir; pickled vegetables such as cornichons, kimchee, poi (taro root), and sauerkraut; and meats such as pemmican. The production of coconut oil was no different.

According to the ancient way, coconut milk was pressed from freshly harvested coconuts and allowed to stand and ferment for up to 36 hours. The brief fermentation time allowed for the coconut water to separate from the less-dense coconut oil. The oil was then collected and gently heated for a brief period in order to evaporate any excess moisture. Finally, it was lightly filtered to remove any solid bits that might remain. The resulting oil was clear and light. It was stable for long periods at high ambient temperatures, and it retained the unique scent, flavor, and health-giving properties of coconut.

Although traditional methods of producing coconut oil had been handed down from generation to generation for many hundreds of years, the knowledge of the process was almost lost due to the convenience afforded by modern industrial edible oil processing. Fortunately for us, however, those traditional methods have survived and are once again being actively passed on and promoted to produce virgin coconut oil today.

Before World War II

Prior to World War II, coconut oil was produced by hand in traditional methods for personal use or as a part of individual families' small cottage industries. In those days, farmers also hulled their own rice by hand. There were no chemical fertilizers, very few doctors, and nothing we consider to be modern conveniences of any kind.

On the other hand, adhering to their indigenous diets made such modern concepts and innovations unnecessary. Plants grew lushly in virgin soil protected by their own naturally inherent defenses. Despite the fact that the sweltering heat and humidity made the potential for parasite, fungal, and bacterial infections high, people stayed well by eating the foods that were naturally suited to growth in that environment.

Tropical inhabitants called for a doctor only in the case of serious traumatic wounds or tropical diseases spread by mosquitoes, such as malaria or dengue fever. It was common for tropical islanders to live robustly into their eighties and nineties without ever having seen a doctor. Chronic debilitating illness was unheard of. The occasional simple illness was treated using a variety of local herbs and coconut oil.

How Did Coconut Oil Get Such a Bad Reputation?

During the earliest part of the twentieth century, coconut oil enjoyed widespread use and tremendous popularity in the burgeoning baking industry of the United States and in the rest of the world as well. Coconut oil's long shelf life and low melting point made it easy to use and keep. And if that had not been enough to hold coconut oil in good graces, it also tastes delicious and smells divine.

In the 1950s, however, research was conducted that seemed to demonstrate that health risks were associated with the consumption of saturated fats. Soon scientists, doctors, and nutritionists informed the general population of these perceived health risks, and by association, coconut oil was labeled as unhealthy. Eventually, it became difficult if not impossible to find coconut oil in the West.

Japanese Occupation of the Pacific

During World War II, the United States lost a rich source of coconut oil when the Japanese occupied the Philippines and other South Pacific islands. The Japanese occupation interrupted the supply for several long years as the war raged on, and coconut oil was no longer available as either a cooking oil or for inclusion in the production of commercial food products.

TO YOUR HEALTH!

Modern vegetable oils are manufactured via a complex succession of industrial processing which begins with crude vegetable oil that has been extracted from its source seed, grain or legume. The crude oil is then degummed, undergoes caustic refining, and is prebleached. Next, it is either dewaxed or hydrogenated and goes through a post-bleaching process. From there it will be either winterized or undergo fractionation, interesterfication and blending. Finally, it will be deodorized because the processing causes rancidity. The final stage of the process before packaging, is either spray-chilling (liquid oils) or plasticization (margarines and shortenings). Alternatively, the deodorized oil may have emulsifiers added to it and begin the refining process again.

—Richard D. O'Brien, *Fats and Oils: Formulating and Processing for Applications*

Because of the shortage in the supply, Western companies worked on creating alternatives to coconut oil, which gave rise to polyunsaturated oils. By the time the war was over, the new polyunsaturated oil industry had made a lot of money. It had begun to actively promote the modern oils, and it was not about to give up its slice of the edible oil market to foreign concerns.

Bad Science

An anti–saturated fat "push" began in the 1950s when it was noted that there had been a sharp rise in heart disease. Yet during the nineteenth century, while people still ate unlimited amounts of butter, eggs, lard, beef, and pork, coronary occlusions (heart attacks) were virtually unknown. The heart attack was not even described in a medical journal until 1912.

Dr. Paul D. White, who was President Eisenhower's personal cardiologist, had not seen his first heart attack until the 1920s, but by the 1950s the incidence of heart disease had risen to account for more than 30 percent of all deaths. So researchers began looking for the cause of this new threat to the nation's health.

Eventually, some researchers suggested that cholesterol levels were the problem and that saturated fats raised cholesterol levels. In one study, the artery plaques found in American soldiers who had died in Korea were examined. Because higher levels of cholesterol were found in arterial plaques, some scientists proposed that cholesterol levels found in foods were also part of the problem.

Soon a "lipid hypothesis" was formed, stating that "saturated fat and cholesterol from animal sources raise cholesterol levels in the blood, leading to deposition of cholesterol and fatty material as pathogenic plaques in the arteries." By the end of the 1950s, saturated fats found in foods were looked upon unfavorably, while new vegetable oils manufactured from corn, soybean, and so on became increasingly popular.

The result was that the new polyunsaturated vegetable oils and hydrogenated vegetable oils were viewed as heart-healthy substitutes for naturally saturated fats. Current research conducted at Harvard, the University of Washington School of Medicine, and elsewhere shows, however, that cholesterol levels in food have little or no effect on blood cholesterol levels. Research published in 2005, in the *Handbook of Experimental Pharmacology* states that, "Based on these studies, the association between dietary cholesterol and CHD (coronary heart disease) risk is, if anything, minor in nature. This is consistent with the finding that an increase in dietary cholesterol intake results in only a minimal increase in the total/high-density lipoprotein cholesterol ratio." Subsequently, the entire lipid theory of heart disease has been summarily rejected by many doctors, and top research scientists have written extensively on the flaws of the "cholesterol theory" of heart disease.

In fact, some who were responsible for the theory itself have even discounted it. In 1997, Dr. Ancel Keys, who is fairly regarded as the father of the cholesterol theory, stated, "There's no connection whatsoever between the cholesterol in food and cholesterol in the blood.

And we've known that all along. Cholesterol in the diet doesn't matter at all unless you happen to be a chicken or a rabbit."

Keys' statement refers to early research that included force-feeding rabbits and chickens with food that was high in cholesterol. Being primarily vegetarian, rabbits and chickens are not physiologically designed for processing huge amounts of cholesterol and as a result, cholesterol levels were raised in their blood. It does not follow, however, that omnivorous humans would experience a similar effect.

TO YOUR HEALTH!

In 1988, Congress held hearings to discuss the safety of tropical oils. Dr. George Blackburn, a Harvard medical researcher, testified that coconut oil has a neutral effect on blood cholesterol, even in situations where coconut oil is the sole source of fat. Surgeon General C. Everett Koop dismissed all the attacks on coconut oil as "Foolishness," and continued by saying, "but to get the word to commercial interests terrorizing the public about nothing is another matter."

—Brian and Marianita Shilhavy, *Virgin Coconut Oil*

Flawed Studies

So what was the cause of the rapid rise in heart disease in early part of the twentieth century? While there are many factors to consider, one factor is that industrialization significantly changed the American diet. Sugary colas were invented in the 1890s. Modern mills began refining grains into white, nutritionally depleted rice, meals, and flours. And in the crucial 60-year period between 1910 and 1970 when coronary heart disease escalated from an unrecognized problem to the cause of death in over 50 percent of our population, this is what occurred in our diet:

- Cholesterol consumption remained unchanged.
- Consumption of refined carbohydrates like sugar, corn syrup, and white flour increased by 60 percent.
- Naturally saturated fat intake dropped significantly.
- The new polyunsaturated and hydrogenated oils replaced natural fats in our diet.

Due to wartime shortages and rationing, butter consumption was declining while the use of vegetable oils, especially oils that had been hardened to resemble butter and lard by hydrogenation, was dramatically increasing. Incredibly, by 1950, butter consumption had dropped from 18 pounds per person per year to just over 10 pounds. Margarine rose from about 2 pounds per person at the turn of the century to 8 pounds. Consumption of vegetable shortening (commonly used in baked goods) remained steady at about 12 pounds per person per year. Manufactured vegetable oil consumption, however, had more than tripled from under 3 pounds per person per year to more than 10 pounds.

The argument can be made that getting less exercise and the increase in fast-food consumption may have been an important contributing factor in the increase in heart disease. But in the period between 1910 and 1970, relatively little had changed in that vein—not in the way things have from 1970 to the present. The first McDonald's restaurant was not established until mid-1940 and the Big Mac didn't debut until 1968. People still worked and played physically hard in 1970, too. Families typically had one car, so people walked and biked more. They had only one TV, no TIVO or VCRs, and no computers—the first home video game system didn't arrive on the scene until May 1972. So entertainment came in the form of fun physical activities, and in 1970, families still ate at home.

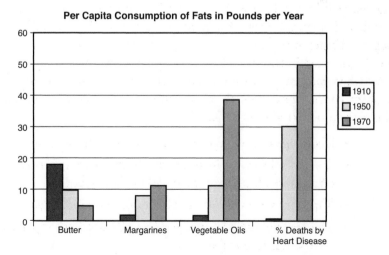

The historical correlation between cholesterol consumption and heart disease rates.

The Edible Oil Industry

Because of its high saturated fat content, coconut oil continued to be vilified by the vegetable oil industry throughout the decades that followed. The soybean industry, in particular, began to condemn the use of all tropical oils. The threat of cheap competition and the millions of dollars the modern oil industry stood to lose required that health and good science take a backseat to profits.

Unfortunately, the tropical oil industries of poorer countries like the Philippines and Indonesia were unable to fight back against the negative smear campaigns of the more wealthy American industrial conglomerates. So for nearly a decade, the scientifically proven health benefits of coconut oil not only remained a secret but were vehemently denied.

Different Types of Coconut Oil

Today there are many different types and brands of coconut oil on the market. These days coconut oil is not only available in health-food stores, but also online and even in supermarkets. Lucky for us! But the labels and names of the products can sometimes seem confusing.

For instance, you might wonder why some coconut oils are so much more expensive than others. Or why some coconut oils don't smell like coconut. Are all coconut oils nutritionally equal? And which coconut oil is the closest to how coconut oil was traditionally made?

Refined Coconut Oil

Most commercial-grade coconut oil is made from *copra*. Copra is the white dried meat of the coconut that most Westerners are familiar with. Copra can be made by sun drying, kiln drying, smoke drying, or a combination of these methods. But when copra is used to make coconut oil, it's not suitable for consumption until it has been refined because most copra is not dried under sanitary conditions.

DEFINITION

Copra, dried coconut meat, is a valuable agricultural product for many coconut-producing countries. Coconut oil can be extracted from copra, and the coconut cake that remains as a by-product of the oil extraction process is used as feed for livestock.

After it has been refined, it is known as RBD coconut oil, which stands for refined, bleached, and deodorized. In the RBD process, the oil is deodorized under high heat, and afterward it is filtered through clays that serve to bleach the oil and remove any impurities. Finally, sodium hydroxide is used to remove any free fatty acids in the interest of prolonging the oil's shelf life.

Some of the more modern RBD refining methods go a step further by using chemical solvents to extract every bit of oil from the copra. Of course, chemical solvents may not mix with your idea of good food, but this method does result in higher yields of oil and increased profits for the producer.

In hot climates where coconut oil remains a liquid all year round, RBD oil is also sometimes hydrogenated or partially hydrogenated to make it solid. In cooler climates, however, there is little reason for doing this because coconut oil will remain solid at temperatures at or below 76°F. (The average annual temperature in tropical climates ranges from 80.3°F to 91.4°F.).

Furthermore, since coconut oil is mostly saturated, there is very little unsaturated oil left to be hydrogenated. (See Chapter 7 for more information on the dangers of hydrogenated trans-fatty acids.) The RBD method is the most commonly used process for mass-producing coconut oil. This oil is very popular for use in cooking and for a variety of other purposes because of its relatively low cost and availability.

RBD oil is an excellent carrier oil for use in toiletry and aromatherapy applications for dry, itchy, or sensitive skin, and it will not clog pores. It is highly valued in the soap-making industry as well because of its resistance to rancidity and its ability to produce a hard soap with a rich, fluffy lather.

Virgin Coconut Oil

Virgin coconut oil can only be extracted from fresh, "noncopra" coconut. High heat and chemicals are not used in the making of virgin coconut oil since the naturally saturated fats in pure coconut oil result in a very stable oil with a shelf life of several years. There are currently two main processes for producing virgin coconut oil:

- In the quick-dry method, fresh coconut meat is quickly dried using minimal heat. Then the meat is pressed, using a mechanical means, and results in the release of the oil.

- In the wet-milling method, the oil is extracted from fresh coconut meat without drying it first. When the meat is pressed, it is *coconut milk* that is released. In the second step of the process, the oil and water are separated using boiling, fermentation, refrigeration, mechanical centrifuge, or enzymes.

 DEFINITION

Coconut milk is the white liquid that results when fresh coconut meat is grated. Its color and rich flavor are due to its high coconut oil content.

The most obvious difference between virgin coconut oil and refined coconut oil is the scent and taste. All virgin coconut oils retain the scent and aroma of coconuts, while copra-based refined coconut oils have no flavor or taste.

Although some grades of refined coconut oil are proclaimed to have coconut flavor, they have not been thoroughly filtered and deodorized, which results in a rather bitter or burnt taste. These grades of refined coconut oil have a shorter shelf life than virgin coconut oil.

Extra-Virgin Coconut Oil

If virgin coconut oil is supposed to be so great, then *extra*-virgin coconut oil must be even better, right? Well, not so fast .... Some manufacturers and retail distributors of virgin coconut oils call their product "extra-virgin coconut oil." But there is no such thing.

There are no processes used to make virgin coconut oil other than the previously mentioned two, so this classification is simply a marketing ploy.

If you see a product labeled "extra-virgin" and it smells and tastes of coconut, it is really virgin coconut oil—and that's a good thing. But don't be fooled. There is no difference between "virgin" and "extra-virgin" coconut oil like there is in the olive oil industry.

Because of the industry's established quality grades, extra-virgin olive oil commands a much higher price than the lower grades of olive oil, which bear the names virgin olive oil, pure olive oil, olive oil, olive pomace oil, or lampante oil.

Unscrupulous marketers try to capitalize on this commonly known fact by labeling their virgin coconut oils as extra-virgin. Don't believe them! When all other things are equal, go with the lower-priced oil.

TO YOUR HEALTH!

In 2004, the journal *Clinical Biochemistry* reported on a study done in India that compared refined coconut oil (CO) to virgin coconut oil (VCO). It found that VCO obtained by the wet process had a beneficial effect in the form of lowered serum lipid components (fats and cholesterol in the blood) as compared to CO.

VCO reduced total cholesterol, triglycerides, phospholipids, LDL and VLDL cholesterol levels, while increasing HDL cholesterol in serum and tissues. The results showed potentially beneficial effects which also included the reduction of LDL oxidation.

—K.G. Nevin and T. Rajamohan, *Clinical Biochemistry*

Expeller-Pressed Coconut Oil

Expeller-pressed coconut oil is a high-quality refined coconut oil. It is the very next best thing to virgin coconut oil. This oil is processed in the old-fashioned way by a process known as physical refining, but it is less expensive than virgin coconut oil.

The modern way of processing coconut oil is by chemical extraction using solvents, which produces higher yields and is less expensive. Expeller-pressed coconut oils, however, do not undergo treatment with chemicals or solvent extracts. Neither are they hydrogenated, so expeller-pressed coconut oils contain no trans-fatty acids. Expeller processing results in a very high-quality, food-grade oil that maintains a high content of healthy medium-chain fatty acids. (See Chapter 5 for more on why these are so important.) This is the common grade of coconut oil that millions of people in Asia consume on a daily basis, where thyroid disease and obesity are still relatively rare.

Expeller-pressed coconut oil is preferred by people who are looking for a bland or tasteless oil because it goes through a steam-deodorizing process that removes the coconut scent and flavor.

The Least You Need to Know

- Coconut oil has always been a healthy, integral part of life among many traditional tropical cultures.
- Before World War II, coconut oil was highly valued worldwide, especially in the baking industry. But then Japanese occupation of the Pacific cut off coconut oil supplies to the rest of the world.
- Bad science and flawed studies convinced the public that even naturally occurring saturated fats were dangerous, paving the way for the modern edible oil industry.
- Coconut oil has returned to the market, and there are several grades from which to choose.

Where Can You Find Coconut Oil?

In This Chapter

- Adding coconut oil to your diet
- Taking coconut oil supplements
- Eating coconut meat as a source of coconut oil
- Finding coconut milk, cream, and flour
- Locating coconut cuisines, foods, and snacks

Health-conscious people and dieters who are trying to increase their intake of coconut oil may be relieved to know that they are not limited to dosing themselves with oil by the tablespoon. Coconut oil can be found in a surprising number of places and forms.

Because of increased demand and modern means of food transportation, people are now able to obtain fresh coconut and related products that were not available to mainlanders only a few years ago. The internet and food-related TV shows, too, have popularized world cuisines and made them accessible in ways they have never been before.

Whether you are interested in simply adding coconut oil directly to your existing diet, designing your own homemade meals around coconut oil products, or looking for ready-made foods that contain appreciable amounts of coconut oil, there are many options today for getting coconut oil into your diet.

Coconut Oil in Pill Form

Some people are interested in coconut oil for its health-promoting properties alone. They are not interested in experimenting with exotic new foods and unfamiliar flavors. All they want to do is get adequate amounts of coconut oil into their bodies in the quickest, most pain-free way possible. If this describes the type of interest you have in coconut oil, you may be hoping that coconut oil pills are available—and they are. But there is a caveat, so please read on before rushing out to buy them.

At the time of this writing, prices range from $14.99 to $25.99 for 120 1,000-milligram gelatin capsules. Those prices don't seem too bad, right? Certainly, they are in line with prices of daily dose multi-vitamin tablets and similar nutritional supplements.

The problem becomes evident upon examining what you actually get for your money in comparison to what the recommended therapeutic dosage is.

A 1,000-milligram coconut oil soft gel capsule is currently the largest one made. Keep in mind that 1,000 milligrams is equal to 1 gram. Most research scientists and doctors who recommend coconut oil as a therapy currently recommend a dosage of between 2 and 3.5 tablespoons per person, per day. Each individual tablespoon is equal to 15 grams. This means that to receive a therapeutic dosage of coconut oil, a person would have to consume an inordinate number of 1,000-milligram capsules. In order to get the recommended amount of coconut oil in capsule form, a person would have to consume between 30 and 52.5 capsules per day!

TO YOUR HEALTH!

Let food be thy medicine, and let medicine be thy food.

—Hippocrates, circa 400 B.C.E.

One must consider the cost as well. Going by the prices previously cited, it would cost between $5.00 and $8.60 per day to keep a person supplied with coconut oil supplements. The same $8.60 could buy a 16-ounce jar of virgin coconut oil that would supply 32 1-tablespoon doses and last approximately 10 days, for a daily cost of about 86 cents. What a savings!

Using jarred virgin coconut oil instead of supplements in capsule form also means you will not have to be concerned with the components of the gel caps themselves, which may contain mineral oil residues from the manufacturing process. Furthermore, many gelatin capsules are derived from beef by-products and may contain growth hormones and antibiotics.

Coconut Meat

The meat of the coconut, which is available in many forms, provides an appreciable amount of coconut oil, and it is also an excellent source of dietary fiber and protein. One 2×2×$\frac{1}{2}$-inch piece of coconut contains 15 grams of coconut oil, about the equivalent of 1 tablespoon.

What sort of coconut meat is best? The easy answer is that fresh is best, but for most people what it comes down to is what kind of coconut is available. Historically speaking, the coconut available to islanders and that which has been available to mainlanders are vastly different in nearly every conceivable way.

While the people of the tropics have always enjoyed the youngest, freshest coconut around, the rest of the world has had to settle for "second best." With increased demand, however, and modern methods of shipping and handling, consumers are beginning to see greater variety in the selection of coconuts available.

Fresh Young Coconut

Young fresh coconut was once something that could only be had while living in or visiting the tropics. When I lived in Hawaii in the 1950s, islanders would not have considered eating any other kind of coconut. Older, brown coconut was "second rate." It was generally used for shredding, packaging, and selling to the rest of the world. These days, however, young green coconut is showing up in supermarkets in many of the larger mainland cities of America. It has special characteristics that make it unique in both taste and usage.

If you live in the tropics and you want a young coconut, you already know what you're looking for—lucky you! But on the mainland, it's not so obvious. A young green coconut will have been trimmed of its outer green husk, leaving a roughly cone-shaped whitish fiber covering. To ensure it remains fresh, the trimmed nut is wrapped in clear plastic and labeled before shipping.

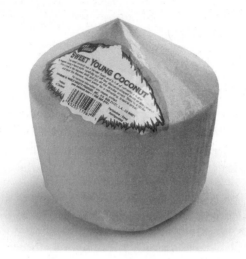

A young coconut as it appears in the supermarket.

Here's how to open a trimmed, young green coconut:

1. Using a strong and heavy knife, like a butcher knife, make an incision by cutting down into the pointed end of the coconut.

2. Next make three more slits to form a square opening on top. This way, you will avoid losing the coconut water inside.

3. Use the knife to pry loose the square plug and access the tender flesh and coconut water.

A young coconut's juice, the coconut water, can be drunk straight from the fruit using a straw. Its flesh should be so tender that it can be scraped from the inside using a spoon. The meat of a young coconut should always be white. Do not eat it if it is pink or any other color because the coconut may have spoiled. A good, fresh young coconut will have clear juice and no sour taste.

Mature Coconut

This is the coconut with which most people are familiar. It is an older nut whose tough outer husk has been completely removed. It is roundish, brown, and hairy in appearance. The nut meat of these coconuts will be quite firm, but it should still have some coconut water inside, so shake before buying.

TO YOUR HEALTH!

Did you know that coconut water was used by Allied Forces during World War II as emergency intravenous fluid for injured or dehydrated troops? Coconut water is normally sterile, and its chemical makeup is very similar to human intracellular fluid.

To open a mature coconut you will need a hammer, a good-sized nail, and a small bath towel.

1. Fold the towel into several thicknesses and place on a firm, sturdy surface.

2. Place the coconut on the towel with its three eyes facing upward.

3. Using the hammer and nail, hammer a hole in each of the coconut eyes. (The shell is a bit softer there.)

4. Drain the coconut water into a cup.

5. When all of the water has drained out, place the coconut back on the towel and give it several sharp whacks with the hammer to break the shell open.

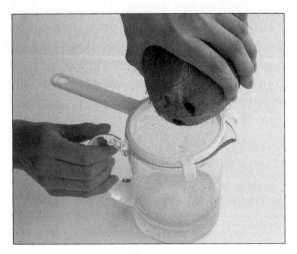

Draining the coconut water.
(Copyright Dorling Kindersley)

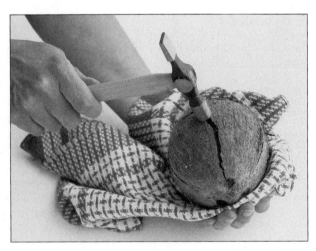

Cracking the coconut.
(Dave King copyright Dorling Kindersley)

The coconut water is good to drink, and the flesh can easily be pried off the shell using a kitchen knife. There will be a thin brown layer of nut meat next to the shell. This layer is part of the coconut meat and is perfectly good to eat.

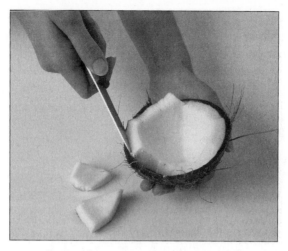

Prying the nutmeat away from the shell.
(Clive Streeter and Patrick McLeavy copyright Dorling
Kindersley)

Copra—Dried and Flaked Coconut

There are several forms of dried coconut. It is essentially the same as
the meat of a mature coconut that has been dried and has undergone
some additional processing. Dried coconut is available in both sweetened and unsweetened forms, in chips, flakes, and finely shredded.

Dried coconut is packaged in a variety of manners as well. The
canned coconut is always more moist than the bagged supermarket
variety, and it is usually more expensive as well. Unsweetened coconut chips and flakes are still most easily found on the internet and
can be bought in 1- to 3-gallon plastic bulk containers that keep the
product viable for very long periods of time.

Coconut Cream and Coconut Cream Concentrate

Commercial coconut creams are usually sold in cans, and the main
ingredient in these products is almost always water. The dietary fiber
of the coconut has usually been stripped out of these commercially
available products as well. So as a general rule, most coconut creams

are not an exceptionally good source of coconut oil. Another thing to be aware of is that almost all commercial coconut creams contain additives that are there to prevent the water from separating from the coconut oil and contain sulfites to keep the product white. Many have added sugar as well.

Coconut cream concentrate is very different from coconut cream, and it is sometimes referred to as coconut butter. It consists entirely of dried coconut meat that has been ground very finely. This means it retains all of the dietary fiber and oil of the coconut and has a creamy consistency similar to other nut butters.

Coconut cream concentrate is a versatile food that many people enjoy spread on bread or crackers. It can be blended into smoothies or stirred into coffee as an alternative to nondairy creamer. It also lends itself as a tasty addition to baked goods and can be used as a base for condiments and sauces. (See Chapters 15 through 17 for more coconut cream concentrate uses and ideas.)

Coconut Milk

Coconut milk is the liquid that exudes from the fresh coconut flesh when it is grated. Its high coconut oil content accounts for the rich taste of the coconut milk.

In tropical traditions, there are two grades of coconut milk: thick and thin.

- Thick milk is made by pressing grated coconut meat to make it release its liquid. Thick milk is used in making desserts and rich sauces.

• To create thin coconut milk, the meat that was pressed in the first process is soaked in warm water and squeezed a second or third time. Thin milk is generally used in soups and lighter cooking applications.

Commercially, coconut milk can be found readily on supermarket shelves packaged in cans (thick) and in cartons in the dairy section (thin).

TROPICAL TIP

You can make your own coconut milk at home using commercially available grated coconut. Simply soak the coconut in hot milk or water for about 30 minutes. Then squeeze through cheesecloth to extract the milk and healthful aromatic oil. This milk will have approximately 17 percent coconut oil by volume, and if left to sit, it will separate to yield a layer of coconut cream on top.

Coconut Flour

Coconut flour is the ground fiber of the coconut meat after most of the oil has been extracted. Its color is off-white and similar in appearance to unbleached all-purpose wheat flour. The healthiest coconut flours are certified organic, unsweetened, and have not been treated with sulfites. Coconut flour is high in dietary fiber and protein and is naturally gluten free.

Coconut flour contains over 19 percent nongluten protein. It makes a great addition to smoothies when extra fiber and protein are desirable. It also makes a healthy thickener for soups and sauces.

Compared to flours made from grains containing gluten proteins, coconut flour has both a higher protein content and a higher fiber content. It can be used to easily augment the fiber content in standard wheat flour recipes by substituting coconut flour for 10 to 30 percent of the wheat flour. Some moist quick-bread recipes can even be made using coconut flour alone. Finally, coconut flour has a natural sweetness about it that allows for a reduction in the amount of sugar used in recipes, while still producing tasty baked goods.

Coconut flour is still not readily available in grocery stores. It can, however, be found in some health-food stores and can be obtained easily online. (See Appendix B for sources.)

Coconut Water

As you might imagine, coconut water does not contain appreciable amounts of coconut oil. It is, however, a healthy component of the coconut. It is the clear liquid found inside fresh young coconut and, to a lesser degree, mature coconut.

Coconut water has long been a popular drink in the tropics. In the Pacific Islands, Southeast Asia, the Caribbean, and some parts of Africa, coconut water is available fresh from street vendors who will open the coconut for the customer on the spot to demonstrate its freshness.

TO YOUR HEALTH!

Did your mom ever tell you that if you accidentally knock out a tooth, you should place it in a glass of milk until you get to a dentist? The milk helps to keep the tooth alive until it can be reimplanted.

Well, according to a study published in the *Journal of Endodontics*, coconut water is even better than milk at keeping a lost tooth alive! Maybe schools should keep a coconut or two handy for times when youngsters accidentally crack their coconuts on the playground.

Elsewhere, coconut water is sold bottled or canned and is marketed as a natural sports or energy drink because its mineral content so closely matches the electrolyte balance that the human body needs.

Coconut Oil in Restaurant Foods

With the burgeoning interest in exotic cuisines, it is becoming much easier to find coconut as a feature of restaurant meals. You just have to know what to look for. Restaurants that feature popular Thai and Indian cuisines are a good place to begin. Other traditional cuisines, such as those of Micronesia, Polynesia, the Caribbean, and Brazil, make good use of coconut, too, but outside of their homelands restaurants with these themes are not as easy to find.

Indian Foods

If you are lucky enough to live near a restaurant that prepares traditional Indian foods, you will have no trouble finding menu items containing coconut products. Indian cuisine is famous for its curries, and that is a splendid place to start, but the cuisine of India offers much, much more.

In India coconut is widely known as *naariyal*, and it is a main ingredient in most of the dishes that originate in the southern region. Southern Indians use coconut oil in cooking their other foods as well, while the rest of India treats coconut mostly as a fruit.

Indians universally employ coconut in the preparation of sweet dishes, and dried coconut is widely used in savory dishes to impart flavor and aroma. Although Indian cuisine is renowned for its distinctive use of herbs and spices, without coconut and coconut oil, many Indian foods would seem relatively flavorless.

The following are some menu items to look for:

- Aviyal, a delightful medley of coconut, hot chiles, and vegetables
- Coconut chikki, a sweetened coconut dessert
- Coconut podi, featuring coconut, red chiles, and black gram (urad dal)
- Vangi ani val, a bean and eggplant side dish
- Achhi ka salan, a fish entrée with distinctly Indian flavors

If you are not fortunate enough to have an Indian restaurant nearby, or if you'd like to try making some Indian coconut recipes on your own, explore the recipes provided in Chapters 15 and 16.

Thai Cuisine

When it comes to coconut in Thai cuisine, soups and curries are definitely the way to go! When dining out Thai style, look for the traditional green curry, *gaeng kiow wan*, which may be made with either chicken, pork, or fish. Panang curry, *gaeng Panang*, and Muslim curry, *gaeng Mussaman*, are two popular chicken or beef dishes.

Among the coconut soups, there is *dom ka gai*, a chicken coconut soup, and *dom ka taleb*, a delicious seafood coconut soup. Here are some other coconut dishes you might find on a Thai menu:

- Kanom krok, a grilled coconut and rice pancake
- Miang kam, a delightful sampler food wrapped in wild pepper or spinach leaves
- Sangkaya, a coconut custard
- Kao niow ma-muang, a coconut "sticky rice" dish
- Coconut ice cream (Yum!)

While not every Thai dish is made with coconut, you will always be able to find a few, and trying them out can be such an adventure. Thai foods are wonderfully full of fresh ingredients, high in antioxidants, and rich in healthy *bioflavonoids*, too. (See Chapter 16 for Thai soup and curry recipes.)

DEFINITION

Bioflavonoids—once known as vitamin P—are naturally occurring plant compounds found in the pigments of fruits and vegetables. Three of the flavonoid classes are ketone-containing compounds that show much promise in preventing and mitigating neurodegenerative disease states such as the various dementias, MS, ALS, and Parkinson's disease.

The Philippines and Polynesia

Unfortunately for North Americans, the cuisines of the Philippines, Polynesia, and Micronesia currently do not seem to hold as much sway among foodies as those of Thailand and India. The result is that there are precious few restaurants devoted to these styles of cooking.

Hawaiian cuisine, however, is unique among the island cuisines because of the history of how other island and Asian cultures assimilated themselves into the native Hawaiian population. These people brought their healthy food traditions along with them and melded them together with Hawaiian traditions to create what we now recognize as Hawaiian cuisine.

Notable among Hawaiian-themed eateries was the grand Hawaii Kai in New York City that reigned among tropical restaurant establishments from 1961 to 1989. Hawaii Kai's menu was exhaustive, running the entire gamut of the vast food culture. If you are fortunate enough to find a Hawaiian restaurant, look for these coconut delicacies that were once faithfully interpreted at Hawaii Kai:

- Dolphinfish (mahi-mahi) simmered in coconut milk
- Haupia, a traditional coconut pudding
- Halakahiki Niu, a pineapple-coconut sauce
- Aloha Lobster, a coconut curry
- Samoan bananas served with coconut cream
- Shrimp Waikiki, a coconut-shrimp tempura

If it turns out you aren't able to find a restaurant that serves these island foods, don't despair. Many of them have been re-created for you in Chapters 15 through 17.

Other Popular Foods and Snacks

With all this talk about exotic cuisines, you might begin to think that they are the only sources for yummy foods that contain coconut oil. Nothing could be further from the truth. Once Westerners discovered coconut, it did not take long before they were inventing their own coconut-based delights. Coconut macaroons are a case in point.

TO YOUR HEALTH!

Eating coconut macaroons to ease symptoms of Crohn's disease is a strange-sounding therapy backed by solid science. People who suffer with Crohn's disease and ulcerative colitis can obtain some relief by eating foods rich in MCTs like coconut oil. One Crohn's patient reported improvement after suffering for 30 years when he began eating just two macaroons each day.

—Brian and Marianita Shilhavy, *Virgin Coconut Oil*

On the other hand, Westerners have tended toward sweet uses for coconut like coconut cakes, coconut cream pies, and candy bars. If you do a little shopping around, though, you will find a good selection of healthier coconut treats available commercially. Oskri Organics makes its Original Coconut Bar that is health food's answer to traditional candy bars. And Orville Redenbacher makes an All in One Coconut Oil Popcorn Kit. Who'd have thought there would ever be theater-style coconut oil popcorn again? Mmmm … I can smell it now!

For real coconut fans who can tolerate a little extra sugar in their diets, a few really old-fashioned treats can still be had as well: the familiar brown, pink, and white Coconut Slice bar by Candy Farm; Maria's pink, green, and white watermelon Coconut Slice bars; and red coconut balls from Hawaii. For sources of these, see Appendix B.

The Least You Need to Know

- Modern methods of shipping have brought young coconuts into mainland supermarkets. The more difficult-to-find items are available in health-food stores and online.
- Buying coconut oil supplements in pill form is not cost effective. It is much more economical to augment coconut oil consumption by incorporating coconut oil or other coconut products—such as tasty coconut meat, milk, cream, and butter—into your food.
- When looking for restaurant meals that feature coconut, think of establishments that showcase Thai and Indian cuisines. Other traditional cuisines—such as those of Micronesia, Polynesia, the Caribbean, and Brazil—make good use of coconut as well.
- Westerners make use of coconut in primarily sweet applications, such as coconut cakes, coconut cream pies, and candy bars. But old-fashioned treats such as Coconut Slice Bars still exist. There are new brands of organic coconut energy bars being made, too, and theater-style popcorn made in coconut oil is finally making a comeback.

What Is the Coconut Oil Diet?

In This Chapter

- Understanding how the diet came about
- Knowing the important contributors
- Working with coconut oil
- Choosing a plan that's right for you

In its simplest form, the coconut oil diet is not really a diet at all. It essentially entails replacing all polyunsaturated oils you use in cooking and all trans-fatty acids in your diet with coconut oil. That's it.

By doing so, you are bound to experience many improvements in health. If you are overweight, you may lose several excess pounds. You will undoubtedly find that your energy level has increased, and you may discover that some minor, but nagging, complaints disappear.

Notable nutritionists, doctors, and health writers, however, have taken this simple concept and built upon it. They have developed full-blown diet plans designed to improve everything from weight loss to Alzheimer's disease. This chapter explores different approaches to the coconut oil diet and how you can design a strategy that is right for you.

Coconut Oil Diets Have Been Around for a While

Of course, the originators of the coconut oil diet were those people of the tropics who naturally ate coconut and used its oil as a staple in their diets as a matter of course. They experienced an enviable degree of health and vitality as long as they adhered to their native diets and did not adopt modern foods and eating habits. In recent years, experts in the fields of health and nutrition have taken this simple concept and expanded on it.

Now there are coconut oil diets that promise to cleanse and detoxify your body. There are coconut oil diets that promise weight loss, improved thyroid function, and increased energy. There is even a coconut oil diet that claims to prevent, halt, or even reverse debilitating and fatal neurodegenerative diseases.

Notable Diets and Authors

The first commercial coconut oil diet was not really a diet at all, but a campaign by Brian and Marianita Shilhavy to promote the not-yet widely known health benefits of coconut oil. Marianita is a certified nutritionist/dietitian and a native of the Philippine islands. She grew up witnessing the excellent health and vitality of her kinsmen who followed the traditional, high-saturated-fat Filipino diet and saw that Filipinos who had adopted modern eating habits suffered.

Marianita and Brian describe in their book, *Virgin Coconut Oil*, how her relatives lived to very advanced ages. One man in particular was over 100 years old and still climbed down Mt. Banahaw and walked to town once a week for market day. Because of the amazing health they witnessed in their rural neighbors, the Shilhavys began to study and use the local medicinal herbs that grew on the mountain.

Over time, the Shilhavys adopted the dietary habits and herbal traditions of their neighbors and eventually began making their own herbal products to market them locally. Brian also became interested in coconut oil because it figured so prominently in the local diet. As he researched the work of lipids expert Dr. Mary Enig, he was astonished to find that coconut oil was a healthy saturated fat that seemed to account for much of the health he saw in the rural Philippines.

To avoid having to use chemically refined (RBD) commercial coconut oil, Brian learned the traditional methods for making virgin coconut oil from the few elders in their community who still possessed that knowledge. The oil was so good and Brian's health improved so much that they began making and marketing coconut oil along with their herbs.

Eventually, the Shilhavys began to receive glowing reports of how people's health had improved since they had begun using the oil. From 2000 until 2004, the Shilhavys did exhaustive research on coconut oil's medium-chain fatty acids and the adverse effects that polyunsaturated fats and trans-fats have on the body. They began reporting their findings in their newsletter and, in 2004, wrote their book *Virgin Coconut Oil: How it has changed people's lives and how it can change yours!* With the publication of that book came the original coconut oil diet.

TO YOUR HEALTH!

"I was diagnosed HIV+ six months ago. I started using VCO [virgin coconut oil] (3 tablespoons, three times a day) two months ago. The viral load went down from 15,500 to 6,000. CD4 count went up from 615 to 705. I am obviously very excited about these results." —Nicola, South Africa

—Brian and Marianita Shilhavy, *Virgin Coconut Oil*

At about the same time, Dr. Bruce Fife published *The Healing Miracles of Coconut Oil* (in 2004, republished by Avery as *The Coconut Oil Miracle*). It was the first book to gather together the pertinent medical research on the health benefits of coconut oil and present it in an understandable format for the general public. Fife's plan recommended optimal dosages of coconut oil that were purported to aid in weight loss, the prevention of heart disease and premature aging, strengthening the immune system, and improving digestion.

Interest piqued and soon thereafter *The Coconut Diet* was written by nutritionist Cherie Calbom, the "Juice Lady." Cherie presented her diet from a cleansing perspective. It employed various detoxification regimens that utilized raw foods and juices while simultaneously incorporating coconut oil into a relatively low-carbohydrate diet. The book cover proclaimed to reveal "the secret ingredient that helps you lose weight while you eat your favorite foods." It especially highlighted the advantages that the medium-chain fatty acids in coconut oil provide for enhanced thyroid function.

Most recently, being a prolific author, Dr. Fife has published the *pièce de résistance* of coconut oil diet books, *Stop Alzheimer's Now!* Based on serious scientific and medical research and copious case studies, this book takes a profound logical leap forward in explaining that, because of its medium-chain fatty acid makeup, coconut oil is an important key to preventing, mitigating, and even reversing chronic and debilitating neurodegenerative disease states—the dementias, multiple sclerosis (MS), Lou Gehrig's disease (ALS), Parkinson's disease, Huntington's chorea, epilepsy, and others. Dr. Fife's book demonstrates the evidence and explains the research that positively links these diseases to diabetes, metabolic syndrome, and insulin resistance in the brain and other nervous tissues.

Can They All Be Right?

Although all of the most notable writers on the health benefits of coconut are correct, their approaches are very different, and the various approaches will not necessarily result in the same positive outcomes. For example, the Shilhavys' approach will benefit anyone, but it would not likely be stringent enough to reverse chronic disease states and may not even be enough to normalize weight in some people.

Cherie Calbom's approach is very healthy indeed, but it might prove problematic for people with diabetes or other metabolic disorders since it relies heavily on juice cleanses and makes use of grains as well. Her plan may provide higher levels of carbohydrate consumption than certain diabetic or hypoglycemic persons can tolerate, making blood-glucose levels erratic and difficult to manage.

Dr. Fife's approach is, by far, the one that will guarantee the most profound results in anyone. Yet it may be too stringent to be tolerated by people who don't sense an urgent need to go to such extreme lengths in the management of their diets.

The answer to which approach is best lies in understanding what your goals are for improving your health and how you stand to benefit from going the extra mile. In the end, the most basic and important aspect of the coconut oil diet is to actually incorporate coconut oil into your diet. To accomplish that, you will need to know some basics about how to handle coconut oil and in what ways it can be used.

How to Work with Coconut Oil

Coconut oil is a very interesting substance. It is comprised of approximately 90 percent saturated fat. Most saturated fats are solid at room temperature—think butter, lard, beef tallow. But coconut oil, because of its unique set of medium-chain fatty acids, has a very low melting point.

At tropical latitudes, coconut oil is a clear liquid all year round. In temperate climates, it is a solid. If you live in a temperate zone or if your home is air conditioned, your coconut oil will be solid most of the time since its melting point is 76°F.

This property of coconut oil is what makes it especially versatile when used in food preparation. When cool, it can be creamed together with sugar or flour as one does when making cookies or pastries. When even minimally warm (normal skin temperature), it liquefies and can be used for pan-frying and sautéing. Coconut oil easily spreads on toast and sandwich bread without tearing holes, yet it firms up to become candy-like under refrigeration.

Proper Storage and Handling

Because of coconut oil's saturated fat content, it is exceptionally stable at relatively high temperatures and does not form free radicals like polyunsaturated fats do. Some oils are so prone to rancidity that they must be kept under refrigeration at all times. Flaxseed oil is an example. But coconut oil's inherent antioxidant properties give it the longest shelf life of any plant oil. Samples of coconut oil that have been held in a constant liquid state, at temperatures above 80°F, for over two years have shown no evidence of breakdown.

There is nothing to prevent you from refrigerating or even freezing coconut oil, though. When coconut oil is cool it is solid and butter-like, and that helps to make measuring small amounts like teaspoons and tablespoons an easy task. Some people like to shape little quenelles of coconut oil, roll them in flaked coconut, and freeze them. The frozen quenelles are like a little candy treat that provides a dose of coconut oil in a highly palatable form.

When measuring coconut oil in large quantities of a cup or more, it is often easier to accomplish if the oil is liquid. To quickly liquefy a jar of coconut oil, you can stand the jar in a shallow pan of simmering water or under a warm running tap. I do not recommend microwaving a jar of coconut oil, however, as it can become dangerously hot very quickly. Furthermore, if the jar is made of a plastic containing BPA (bisphenol A), when you microwave the container it increases the amount of BPA that leaches into your food. BPA is a toxic substance that readily combines with fats and oils.

AW, NUTS!

BPA mimics estradiol, a sex hormone that can cause major changes in your body, including structural damage to the brain, hyperactivity, early puberty, and disrupted reproductive cycles.

Substituting Coconut Oil for Other Oils

If you prefer using coconut oil as a natural addition to your diet rather than dosing by the spoonful, you will want to know how to use it in the course of normal meal preparation. This is how it has been traditionally used in the tropics.

Generally speaking, coconut oil can be substituted in equal amounts for any fat or oil called for in a recipe. For instance, if you are to sauté a cup of onions in 2 tablespoons of cooking oil, use 2 tablespoons of coconut oil instead. Coconut oil can be used to grease baking pans, to brush on roasting meats to brown them in the oven, in baking recipes, etc.

The only major concern with regard to substituting coconut oil comes with frying. Different oils have different smoke points. So if you are accustomed to pan-frying a food at 400°F, you may have to make a temperature adjustment. As you can see in the following table, virgin coconut oil reaches its smoke point at 350°F.

Comparative Smoke Points of Fats

Fat	Quality	Smoke Point (°F)
Butter	–	250–300
Canola	Expeller	375–450
Canola	High oleic	475
Canola	Refined	400
Coconut	Virgin	350
Coconut	Refined	450
Corn	Refined	450
Lard	–	370
Olive	Extra-virgin	375
Olive	Virgin	391
Olive	Extra-light	450
Soybean	Refined	460
Shortening	–	360
Sunflower	Refined	440

Adjusting the temperature downward will likely mean that the fry time will need to be increased, which may or may not yield the quality finish to which you are accustomed. Frying is an area that requires a little bit of experimentation in order to become proficient.

AW, NUTS!

Never heat oil beyond its smoke point. Doing so causes breakdown of the fat and may result in the oil spontaneously combusting into flames.

Matching the Oil to the Food

Another consideration when substituting coconut oil for other oils is flavor and aroma. Virgin coconut oil retains a slight coconut flavor and quite a lot of the fragrance of coconut.

The flavor and fragrance of coconut may be desirable when substituting coconut oil for other fats in a dessert recipe. Virgin coconut oil perfectly complements the unique flavors of Thai and Indian cuisine as well. But for some people, it can be disconcerting to stare at a breakfast plate of eggs over-easy and smell warm coconut instead. It's as if the brain is getting mixed signals because it's not accustomed to associating certain aromas with certain foods.

I can tell you that there is nothing wrong with using virgin coconut oil to fry eggs or to make grilled cheese sandwiches. The taste remains the same as it always has because the flavors of most foods are distinct and more assertive than that of the oil—especially when it is used in small amounts. There is, however, an initial surprise when you encounter the coconut fragrance.

To get around the aroma, if that is a problem, simply use expeller-pressed or RBD coconut oil. Both are flavorless and fragrance-free oils, and they both have a higher smoke point, too.

Working with Other Coconut Products

Coconut oil is a component of every coconut product except coconut water. Due to the high-heat stability of coconut oil, most coconut products can be held at room temperature, in sanitary conditions, for very long periods of time. The higher the percentage of coconut oil in a product, the longer it will remain fresh.

Therefore, coconut butter (coconut cream concentrate), having an extremely high coconut oil content, can be stored in a jar at room temperature almost indefinitely—much like peanut butter.

Coconut cream concentrate, however, is very stiff at room temperature and is rock solid under refrigeration. To measure any quantity of coconut cream concentrate, it is almost necessary to warm it up a bit. Placing the jar in a simmering pot of water for a few minutes usually will make it much easier to scoop out and measure.

Coconut butter is delicious spread on bread. I especially enjoy a teaspoon added to a mug of hot cocoa or coffee. Don't be alarmed if you detect a few drops of oil floating on top of your beverage, though. It may look a little strange, but it tastes divine.

Canned coconut milk and coconut cream have a lower percentage of oil than coconut butter. They will remain liquid at room temperature and mostly liquid even under refrigeration. Once a can of coconut milk or coconut cream has been opened, any unused portion should be stored in a closed container in the refrigerator and used within a few days.

Commercial coconut milk and coconut cream are versatile products that can be added to soups, stews, and sauces in the same way you might use dairy products. Freshly made coconut milk should never be boiled, though, because boiling may cause your sauce to break—the fat and water will separate, resulting in a curdled appearance.

Flaked coconut is very moist if bought in a can. To maintain the freshness and moisture of bagged flaked coconut, immediately transfer any unused portion to a glass canning jar and store in the refrigerator or freezer. Storing flaked coconut in plastic containers allows the plastic to absorb some of the precious coconut oil, and some plastic bags allow moisture, in the form of water, to evaporate as well. Flaked and grated coconut are excellent as decorative garnishes, as an addition to cereals and baked goods, and as a high-fiber filler for meatballs and some stuffings.

Like sugar and grain-based flours, coconut flour is attractive to common pantry critters and should be stored in a sealed container in a cool, dry place. If stored properly, coconut flour will remain fresh at room temperature for about one year. To use coconut flour in baking, simply substitute 10 to 30 percent coconut flour for the flour called for in the recipe.

Different Diets for Different Reasons

Now that you are familiar with various coconut products and how to handle them with finesse, you are ready to embark on the coconut oil diet that best suits you. As previously mentioned, even if you do nothing else, adding coconut oil to your diet will result in improved health and energy. Yet people with specific goals or serious health concerns will benefit much more by selecting a coconut oil diet plan that focuses on their particular needs.

- If you are young and have no known health problems, the easiest way to approach the coconut oil diet is as the Shilhavys propose. This approach is outlined in the section titled "For Normal Health and Maintenance."

- If your major concern is significant weight loss and getting blood pressure and cholesterol into normal ranges, you will be interested in the section titled "For Weight Loss the Low-Carb Way."

- If you have no blood-sugar issues (either high or low) and are interested in a cleansing and detoxification program along with adding coconut oil to your diet, the section "For Cleansing and Improved Health" may be for you.

- Finally, if you have any serious health concerns—such as diabetes, Alzheimer's disease, another dementia, MS, cardiovascular disease, etc.—or you are seriously interested in prevention, the section "For Serious Conditions and Health Concerns" is for you.

For Normal Health and Maintenance

This is the easiest plan to implement, but depending on your motivation, it can also be the most radical dietary change of the four plans. In the interest of normal health and maintenance, you will have three goals to keep in the forefront of your mind:

- Replace all polyunsaturated oils and all hydrogenated fats (trans-fats) in your diet with coconut oil.

- The only other recommended cooking oils include red palm oil and butter from organically raised, grass-fed beef. Extra-virgin olive oil may be consumed but should not be heated as is done in cooking.

- Consume the equivalent of 2 to 3 tablespoons of coconut oil daily. This can come in the form of other coconut products, but you will have to consider each product's conversion factor.

This is a very easy and straightforward approach to the coconut oil diet, and if this is all you do, you will undoubtedly reap the benefits of improved health. What you may not have considered, however, is how numerous the sources of polyunsaturated fats and trans-fats are. They don't just reside in the cooking oil bottles and shortening cans of your pantry. They are everywhere.

To take this dietary approach to the next level, you will need to take inventory of your pantry, refrigerator, and freezer.

Polyunsaturated fats and trans-fats are in nearly every processed food product. Even snack foods with bright, eye-catching sunburst labels that proclaim "0g Trans-Fat!" contain trans-fat. Here is how you will know: read every ingredient on each food product's label.

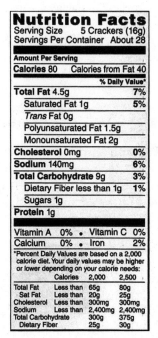

Nutrition facts label for a box of crackers.

Near the nutrition facts label on packaged foods you will find an ingredients list. The ingredients list for these crackers looks like the following:

> **INGREDIENTS:** Unbleached enriched flour, sugar, soybean oil, partially hydrogenated cottonseed oil, sea salt, salt, malted barley flour, baking soda, yeast.

Near the middle of this ingredients list, you will read, *"partially hydrogenated* cottonseed oil." Anytime you see the word *hydrogenated* or the term *partially hydrogenated* in an ingredient list, there are trans-fats in the food. Even if the nutrition facts label states "Trans-Fat 0g" or lists no value, as this label does. The sneaky way food manufacturers get around this sticky problem is by reducing the serving size.

For instance, if the serving size were 3 pieces, the trans-fat content in that amount of food might measure 2 grams trans-fat. But if the manufacturer arbitrarily decides to reduce the serving size to 1 piece, suddenly there is less than 1 gram of trans-fat per serving. This allows manufacturers to state that there are 0 grams trans-fat or none. Be aware, however, that less than one does not mean none.

So to go the whole distance with this dietary plan, you must become a label reader. Hydrogenated fats will be hiding in boxed, bagged, canned, and bottled foods of nearly every kind. Salad dressings, baked goods, breaded products, condiments, and snacks are some of their very favorite hiding places.

For Weight Loss the Low-Carb Way

The late Dr. Robert C. Atkins of the *New Diet Revolution* fame got it right. Although he does not specifically recommend using coconut oil in his book, it fits beautifully into his diet. Dr. Atkins, a cardiologist, advocated a low-carbohydrate ketogenic diet for maintaining ideal weight, correcting metabolic disorders, preventing heart and vascular disease, reducing blood pressure and blood-glucose levels, and killing off pesky yeast infections.

What does not fit is the use of soy products, which are harmful to thyroid health, and his allowance of polyunsaturated and trans-fats.

Essentially, the ideal low-carbohydrate diet would do the following:

- Allow all whole meats, poultry, seafood, and eggs.
- Allow all healthy fats, including liberal amounts of coconut oil.
- Allow amounts of all raw or cooked vegetables that remain under a certain level of carbohydrate content.
- Eliminate all sugars.
- Eliminate all grains, starches, and sweet fruits until the body has nearly achieved its goal weight and blood chemistries—working them back into the diet very gradually as long as no adverse reactions or weight gain result.
- Eliminate or severely restrict alcohol.

As with the previous plan, special attention needs to be given to label reading. Sugars and trans-fats lurk everywhere. Reliance on whole foods over processed manufactured foods and vigilance in reading labels are the keys to success.

For Cleansing and Improved Health

Cherie Calbom's approach to the coconut oil diet is more involved than the previous two plans, and it may not be suitable for certain people who have blood-sugar disturbances. It certainly is the least carbohydrate restrictive of the diet plans.

- This plan encourages the consumption of healthy fat—so coconut oil is "in" (2 to 3 tablespoons per day) and polyunsaturates and trans-fats are "out."
- It is also a relatively low-carbohydrate diet that eliminates refined grains, potatoes, sugar, desserts, and alcohol.
- It emphasizes antioxidant-rich vegetables. Generally speaking, this means the brightly colored ones: beets, carrots, dark leafy greens, and peppers.
- It favors lean proteins over fatty meats. Think chicken or turkey breast (no skin) and broiled or poached fish.

There are four phases in this approach. Phase I is the most stringent aspect of the program. It lasts 21 days. During that time, you would consume 2 to 3 tablespoons of virgin coconut oil per day. The only other oil allowed is extra-virgin olive oil.

During this period, lean fish, chicken, turkey, lamb, and beef are allowed, along with eggs, limited amounts of nuts, and goat cheese. Eight to ten glasses of water are consumed, and caffeinated beverages like coffee are avoided.

Phase II is a cleansing period. This is the phase that many diabetics and hypoglycemics may not be able to tolerate. The Colon Cleanse is an ongoing process that may take as many as eight weeks. These cleansing days are full of raw juices, fiber shakes, raw vegetable salads, and probiotic supplements.

The Liver Cleanse is a seven-day plan that emphasizes raw juices, herbal teas, and a carrot/lemon/olive oil salad. No animal proteins are consumed during the liver cleanse. The Gallbladder Flush is similar to the Liver Cleanse. It also runs for seven days and eliminates animal proteins.

Finally, the Kidney Cleanse is a seven-day plan that works to reduce inflammation and remove excess uric acid from the body. It relies heavily on herbal teas, light (mostly vegetarian) soups and stews, salads, and raw vegetables.

Phases III and IV introduce new carbohydrates at a rate that should prevent weight gain until finally the dieter reaches a comfortable, stable weight. At this point, the general diet is adhered to for life, and the cleanses are repeated periodically.

For Serious Conditions and Health Concerns

The coconut oil diet as proposed by Dr. Bruce Fife effectively takes the dieter back to the level and balance of macronutrients for which the body is ideally suited—the diet that Pacific Islanders and other traditional peoples consumed before being Westernized. It provides ketone therapy (you'll learn more about ketones in Chapter 9) in the form of a ketogenic diet that benefits the body's various organs and systems and has been successfully used in the treatment of epilepsy for 90 years. In addition to reducing or eliminating seizures, this same diet has proven benefits for those who suffer from Alzheimer's, Huntington's, or Parkinson's disease, other dementias, MS, ALS, and diabetes.

- The first step in this diet is to raise ketone levels. This is accomplished by consuming at least 5 tablespoons of coconut oil every day—2 at breakfast time and the remaining 3 at other intervals during the day.

- A standard low-carb diet is followed, allowing between 25 and 100 grams of carbohydrates per day. The number of carbs allowed is determined by the dieter's fasting blood-sugar score. If that number is not known, the 25-gram carb rule is followed.

- Dental hygiene is an important part of this program, including oil pulling therapy, which is based in *Ayurvedic medicine* and uses coconut oil orally as a cleanser and to enhance immune function. (See Chapters 13 and 18 for more on oil pulling.)

- Dr. Fife recommends dietary supplements for people who are experiencing neurodegenerative disease: an iron-free multivitamin, alpha-lipoic acid (ALA), coenzyme Q10 (ubiquinol), magnesium, vitamin C, L-carnitine, and curcumin.

- Other recommendations include adding red palm oil to the diet, including 4 to 8 ounces of fish per week as a source of DHA, getting adequate vitamin D through sun exposure or by supplementation, and exercising regularly as tolerated.

DEFINITION

Ayurvedic medicine (or Ayurveda) is one of the world's oldest medical
systems. It was developed in India and has evolved over thousands of
years. The term "Ayurveda" is comprised of the Sanskrit words *ayur* (life)
and *veda* (science or knowledge)—literally meaning, "the science of
life." In the West, Ayurvedic medicine is considered a complementary
medical system because it evolved apart from modern allopathic
medicine. Ayurveda employs the use of herbs and specially tailored
diets and techniques designed to balance the body, mind, and spirit.

Dr. Fife maintains that the diet should consist mostly of whole, fresh,
and organically grown foods, including animal proteins, full-fat
dairy (raw if possible), nuts, low-starch vegetables, and fruits. At
the same time, prepackaged and processed foods should be avoided
because they contain additives and preservatives such as trans-fats,
nitrites, nitrates, MSG, aspartame, iron (ferrous sulfate), aluminum
salts and compounds, hydrolyzed vegetable protein (soy), soy protein
isolate, and "natural flavor," which should be eliminated.

Water is the drink of choice. Sugars, corn syrup, and refined or
synthetic sweeteners should be completely eliminated. The only
acceptable oils are coconut, palm, olive, and macadamia nut oil.

The Least You Need to Know

- The coconut oil diet replaces all polyunsaturated fats and
  trans-fats in the diet with coconut oil.
- Dr. Bruce Fife, Cherie Calbom, Dr. Robert C. Atkins, and Brian
  and Marianita Shilhavy have made important contributions
  toward making the coconut oil diet a viable dietary plan for
  people with a variety of needs and goals.
- Coconut oil is easily worked into the diet by a straight 1:1
  substitution of coconut oil for other oils. Coconut flour can
  substitute from 10 to 30 percent of the wheat flour called for
  in most baking recipes.
- Once you have defined your health goals, it is easy to choose
  a coconut oil diet plan that suits your needs.

The Science Behind Coconut Oil

Part

2

What makes coconut oil so healthy?

In recent years, that has been the question on the minds of many scientists, doctors, and nutritionists—and they have been busy finding the answers! You will find them, too, in Part 2 of this book.

We explore the unique makeup of coconut oil and how its special fatty acids work in providing coconut oil's many healthy benefits. Each of coconut oil's fatty acids provides different advantages. Each one is described, as well as the antioxidant, antiviral, antibacterial, and anti-inflammatory properties of medium-chain triglycerides (MCTs). Countless interesting studies inform the important dietary role played by naturally saturated fats. These studies and their findings are discussed from both a historic and modern perspective. Finally, we compare and contrast coconut oil with other dietary fats and oils, explaining what the outcome of using each fat is, which fats are healthy for cooking purposes (and why), and how you can know the difference.

What Makes Coconut Oil So Healthy?

In This Chapter

- Knowing the facts about fats
- Understanding coconut oil's special MCTs
- Discovering antioxidant, anti-inflammatory, and antimicrobial qualities

In 1977, official public health recommendations to reduce fat intake were made for the U.S. population (especially adults) by the U.S. Senate Select Committee on Nutrition and Human Needs. The public was advised to keep total fat consumption to less than 30 percent of calories. The idea was that if total fat consumption was reduced, it would necessarily reduce the amount of saturated fat consumed—and saturated fat was thought to be linked to increased volumes of LDL (bad) cholesterol in the bloodstream.

All of this was based on epidemiologic data, which suggested that elevated cholesterol increased the risk of heart disease. Practically speaking, however, it is impossible to achieve an adequate diet without the inclusion of saturated fat. And nutritionally speaking, it is ill advised to try. This chapter explores how the particular saturated fats found in coconut oil are desirable components of a healthy diet.

Medium-Chain Triglycerides (MCTs)

All dietary fats are molecules made up of carbon atoms linked in chains. Primarily because of official recommendations to reduce saturated fat consumption, the main form of fat consumed in the American diet is long-chain triglycerides (LCTs), which range from 14 to 18 carbons in length.

On the other hand, medium-chain triglycerides (MCTs), like those found in coconut oil, range from 6 to 12 carbons in length. In capric acid, shown in the following figure, C 10:0 means 10 total carbon atoms and no double bonds. The absence of double bonds indicates total saturation of carbons with hydrogen.

Capric Acid (C 10:0):

Capric Acid

Oleic Acid (C 18:1):

Oleic Acid

The structural differences in medium-chain and long-chain triglycerides.

The shorter chain length of MCT fats in coconut oil imparts unique properties that enhance human health. One of these properties is that MCTs are absorbed intact and delivered directly to the liver to be used for energy. Other types of dietary fats must be broken down in the small intestine and transformed into another type of fat before entering the bloodstream and being transported to where they can be utilized. Coconut oil is composed of mostly medium-chain saturated fatty acids.

Saturated Fatty Acid Composition: One Fluid Ounce of Coconut Oil

Lipid (Fat) Component	Amount	By Volume
C 6:0 Caproic acid	168 mg	0.69%
C 8:0 Caprylic acid	2,100 mg	8.7%
C 10:0 Capric acid	1,680 mg	6.9%
C 12:0 Lauric acid	12,488 mg	52%
C 14:0 Myristic acid	4,705 mg	20%
C 16:0 Palmitic acid	2,296 mg	9.5%
C 18:0 Stearic acid	784 mg	3.2%

USDA Publication: SR21

By far, the major MCT component of coconut oil is lauric acid at 52 percent by volume. Lauric acid plays a very special role in nutrition, and outside of mother's milk, coconut oil is the best source. Lauric acid and the other MCTs in coconut oil will be discussed next.

Lauric Acid and Monolaurin

A problem that has become global in scale when it comes to treating infections caused by numerous organisms is antibiotic resistance. Antimicrobials that are safe and effective and do not promote resistance are greatly needed.

Monolaurin is recognized as being a highly antimicrobial natural substance that has been extensively researched for its potential use in the food processing and manufacturing industry. Monolaurin is a monoester formed from lauric acid, which has profound antiviral and antibacterial activity. A monoester is in a class of chemical compounds formed by the bonding of an alcohol and an organic acid, with the loss of one water molecule for each ester group formed. Fats are esters, produced by the bonding of fatty acids with the alcohol, glycerol. The antimicrobial activity of the monoglyceride of lauric acid has been recognized and reported since 1966.

Lauric acid has received a bit less attention than monolaurin because it exists as a natural component of foods and cannot be patented. Therefore, relatively little funding has been made available for its research.

While monolaurin is many times more biologically active than lauric acid in killing viruses and bacteria, lauric acid is converted to monolaurin in the body. Unfortunately, the rate and mechanism of this conversion is not yet well understood. These medium-chain fatty acids are unique in their antimicrobial activity in that other fats (like diglycerides and triglycerides) have no effect against pathogenic microorganisms.

So how do lauric acid and monolaurin do their magic? Research (a large body of which is credited to Jon J. Kabara, BS, MS, PhD) has suggested that monolaurin accomplishes its virucidal and bactericidal effects by dissolving the lipid envelopes of pathogens. Another antimicrobial effect seems to be the way these MCTs interfere with signals that would normally direct the cells to replicate themselves.

Lauric Acid Content in Foods

Food	Amount per Cup
Coconut cream, raw	37.0 grams
Coconut cream, canned	23.3 grams
Fresh grated coconut, packed	19.4 grams
Fresh grated coconut, loose	11.9 grams
Granola (with coconut oil and coconut)	6.05 grams
Coconut cream pudding	1.29 grams
Whole milk	0.23 grams

U.S. Department of Agriculture Handbooks, nal.usda.gov/ref/ USDApubs/aghandbk.htm

Myristic Acid

Myristic acid is a saturated, 14-carbon fatty acid occurring in most animal and vegetable fats, particularly butterfat and coconut, palm, and nutmeg oils, and it is sometimes used in the food industry as a flavoring agent. Many Westerners consume very little myristic acid, however, because this fatty acid is found primarily in coconut oil and dairy fats, which many people avoid. Myristic acid is an important fatty acid that the body uses to stabilize many different proteins, including proteins that are integral to a properly functioning immune system.

Palmitic Acid

Palmitic acid is so named because it was first isolated from palm oil in the mid-1800s. In 2010, a Korean study found that palmitic acid does possess antioxidant properties, and it was shown to aid in the prevention of atherosclerosis in rats. Palmitic acid was once thought to raise blood levels of cholesterol, but in fact, it has been shown to reduce cholesterol and reduce the need for insulin, too. Osteopathic physician Dr. Joseph Mercola, who focuses on a preventative approach to health, mentions palmitic acid being especially useful in the prevention of *metabolic syndrome*.

DEFINITION

Metabolic syndrome is the name for a cluster of risk factors that increase the risk for coronary artery disease, type 2 diabetes, and stroke.

Caprylic Acid

Caprylic acid is another MCT that is found in both coconut oil and mother's milk. It has the wonderful ability to kill yeast overgrowth in the gut and thereby reduce or eliminate systemic yeast infection. According to the *Physicians' Desk Reference Guide to Nutritional Supplements*, caprylic acid may also have a beneficial effect on high blood pressure.

It seems that Crohn's disease patients may benefit from caprylic acid as well. A study conducted by a team of Japanese researchers at Chiba University's Graduate School of Medicine found that caprylic acid suppresses IL-8 secretion by Caco-2 cells, which is in part responsible for the inflammatory intestinal disease.

Capric Acid

Capric acid also has strong antiviral and antimicrobial properties. In the body, capric acid is converted into monocaprin, which aids in defending against and eradicating harmful viruses, bacteria, and yeast. Because capric acid is an MCT, it is quickly transported to the liver for an instant source of energy as well.

A joint study published in the *American Journal of Clinical Nutrition* in 2008 shows that, in fact, MCT consumption actually may increase energy expenditure, leading to the loss of excess weight. And in Iceland, researchers reported in 2006 that monocaprin even makes a good denture disinfectant!

Stearic Acid

In 1994, Tine Tholstrup and colleagues published in the *American Journal of Clinical Nutrition* that fats high in stearic acid favorably affect blood lipids (cholesterol) and "factor VII coagulant activity." In other words, they proclaimed that stearic acid is a heart-healthy fat. There is not a large percentage of stearic acid in coconut oil—beef and cocoa are better sources—but when it comes to having a healthy heart, every little bit counts.

Caproic Acid

Caproic acid is also one of the MCT saturated fatty acids found in coconut oil, although it constitutes the smallest portion of MCT fat by volume. It is useful in metabolizing other fats and is used therapeutically in special diets for patients with fat-malabsorption syndromes.

Antioxidant Properties

Recently, considerable interest has developed around the *antioxidant* properties of food. Numerous studies suggest that the consumption of foods containing dietary *phenols* may significantly contribute to human health. Olive oil is one of the edible oils known for its high phenolic content.

Although not attributable to its MCT content, coconut oil also contains considerable antioxidant phenolic properties. It is interesting to note, however, that according to research conducted at Putra University in Malaysia, virgin coconut oil has shown greater proven beneficial effects than RBD coconut oil in clinical trials that examined antioxidant potential. (See Chapter 2 for more information on virgin and RBD coconut oil.)

DEFINITION

Antioxidants are substances that reduce damaging oxidation by free radicals. Well-known antioxidants include vitamins C and E. Antioxidants reduce the risk of cancer and the development of age-related diseases.

Phenols are chemical compounds found in plants that contain protective antioxidants to help defend the body against free radical damage and chronic illnesses.

The study concluded that the RBD process destroys some of the oil's biologically active components, like its phenolic compounds. Since then, a number of studies have confirmed the higher phenolic content in virgin coconut oil. This would correlate with its higher antioxidant activity.

Antiviral and Antibacterial Properties

According to Dr. Bruce Fife, coconut oil has been widely used for its actions against viruses, bacteria, and yeast in many places throughout the world. In India, it is still an important ingredient in the tradition of Ayurvedic medicine, which has been practiced for thousands of years and still is the primary medicine for millions of people. The people in Panama will drink coconut oil by the glassful to recover from illness, and in Jamaica it is used as a heart tonic.

While the general population in the West is still mostly unaware of the therapeutic properties of coconut oil, these properties are well known to scientists who specialize in lipid research. The MCT fats in coconut oil are used in hospitals for feeding patients who have problems with digestion or fat absorption, and in the care of premature infants and of those who are unable to digest other fats. It is even a primary ingredient in many commercially available infant formulas.

Studies show that the lauric acid in coconut oil is effective against deadly antibiotic-resistant *Staphylococcus aureus* (MRSA). Monolaurin also inhibits production of *staphylococcal toxic shock toxin-1*, which results in TSS (toxic shock syndrome), a rare but serious infection that can affect either males or females, but especially during adolescence.

The staph bacteria that is responsible for TSS, and many others, have begun to mutate into pathogens that are resistant to conventional treatment with antibiotic therapies, and medicine is rapidly running out of viable treatment options. The studies of monolaurin's ability to disable bacteria without stimulating them to develop resistance may provide an important clue to the development of effective new treatment therapies.

TO YOUR HEALTH!

According to research published in 1998 and 1999 by Mary G. Enig, PhD, lipid-coated bacteria inactivated by monolaurin include the following:

- *Helicobacter pylori*, responsible for gastric (stomach) ulcers
- *Hemophilus influenzae* (Hib), seen especially in toddlers
- *Listeria monocytogenes*, responsible for food poisoning
- *Staphylococcus aureus* and deadly MRSA
- *Streptococci* groups A, B, F, and G, including *Streptococcus agalactiae*, which causes sepsis in newborns

The results of one study are particularly exciting. In this trial, 15 HIV+ patients were compared at the following dosage levels: 2.4 grams monolaurin, 7.2 grams monolaurin, and 50 milliliters coconut oil. The object of the study was to discover whether the patients' viral load could be reduced. After six months, one patient's viral load was too low to measure, and he was not included in the final statistics. Seven patients had reduced viral loads at their three-month check, and eight patients showed reduced viral loads by the six-month check. Most interesting, though, is that only three of the patients had "significant" reductions. One of those was taking the low-dose monolaurin. The other two were taking the coconut oil.

Other lipid-encapsulated viruses that are inactivated by monolaurin include:

- Cytomegalovirus and Epstein-Barr virus, which cause mononucleosis
- Herpes simplex types 1 and 2, responsible for cold sores and genital herpes
- Herpes varicella zoster, the virus responsible for chicken pox and shingles
- Human immunodeficiency virus, HIV-1, HIV+
- Human T-lymphotropic virus type 1, adult T-cell lymphoma
- Influenza virus, the flu
- Rubella, the German measles virus
- Pneumonovirus, a respiratory virus affecting humans, cattle, sheep, and cats
- Respiratory syncytial virus, which causes cold and flu–like symptoms
- Rubeola, the red measles virus

In addition to coconut oil's ability to fight bacteria and viruses, a number of fungi, yeasts, and protozoa are inactivated or killed by lauric acid, too. These fungi include several species of ringworm, *Candida albicans*, and the protozoan parasite *Giardia lamblia*.

Anti-Inflammatory Properties

It logically follows that if coconut oil is able to disable and kill pathogenic viruses, bacteria, and parasites, the associated *inflammation* would also be reduced as a secondary effect. One study, however, showed direct anti-inflammatory properties in coconut oil.

DEFINITION

Inflammation is a condition recognized by the presence of heat, pain, reddened tissue, and swelling.

This study, conducted in Thailand and published in *Pharmaceutical Biology* in 2010, looked at some of the pharmacological properties of virgin coconut oil. The natural pure oil from coconut milk was prepared without using chemical or high-heat treatment.

Rats were subjected to various means of inducing inflammation, which resulted in edema (swelling) of the rats' ears and paws, writhing, and fever. The anti-inflammatory, analgesic, and antipyretic effects of virgin coconut oil were assessed by observing that virgin coconut oil caused a reduction in ear and paw swelling, a reduction in pain that was evidenced by a reduced writhing response, and an antipyretic effect (fever reduction).

The Least You Need to Know

- The official recommendations for people to reduce fat consumption across the board were ill conceived and resulted in the elimination of healthy saturated fats from many diets.

- Coconut oil possesses an array of unique medium-chain saturated fatty acids that support immunity and resistance to various disease-causing pathogens, including viruses, bacteria, yeasts, and parasites.

- Coconut oil destroys the lipid covering of viruses and bacteria and disrupts their ability to replicate.

- Coconut oil is antiviral, anti-inflammatory, antibacterial, and antioxidant.

- The phenolic compounds in coconut oil have substantial antioxidant action in the body, and virgin coconut oil has greater antioxidant potential than does refined coconut oil.

- Coconut oil has been proven to have an anti-inflammatory effect beyond that which can be attributed to its ability to enhance immunity.

What Studies Show About Coconut Oil

Chapter

6

In This Chapter

- Realizing that natural diets are high-fat diets
- Making skinny pigs and fat people
- Using fats for energy, weight control, immunity, and brain function

Have you ever wondered what a high-fat diet in the United States in the late nineteenth and early twentieth century looked like? It was primarily made up of butter, eggs, whole milk and cheeses, and animal fats. Even the margarines of that time were made from animal fats such as lard and tallow or the saturated fats from coconut oil and palm oil. These high-fat diets, which at that time were considered to be healthy, were rich in saturated fats. In fact, in those days doctors often prescribed high-fat diets as a part of their treatments for serious diseases.

Today the world has witnessed a drastic reduction in the consumption of saturated fats, but this change has not brought about the expected reduction in health problems. In fact, statistics show that obesity rates and other chronic disease states are at all-time highs. The much-touted low-fat dictum is rapidly losing credibility, and this chapter explores what place naturally saturated fats like coconut oil should have in a healthy diet.

Saturated Fats in Traditional Diets

In science, fats and oils are known as lipids. Lipids that are liquid at room temperature are called oils, and those that are solid are fats. In nature, fats are nearly ubiquitous—they are everywhere. Fats are found in animal sources in the form of tallow and lard; in fish and other marine animals; in vegetables and fruits like olives, avocados, and coconut; in nuts, seeds, and legumes such as walnuts, sesame seeds, peanuts, and soybeans; and in whole grains like wheat and corn. A diet that is rich in natural foods will naturally be high in fat. Dietary fats are essential—without them we cannot survive.

TO YOUR HEALTH!

Botanically speaking, a coconut is a fibrous one-seeded drupe. Drupes are fruits that have a hard, stony covering enclosing the seed, like peaches and olives have. The name derives from the word *drupa,* which means "overripe olive."

Because our ancestors ate natural foods, their diets were naturally high in fat, too. There is a common misconception that the animals our ancestors ate had flesh that was lower in saturated fat than that which is found in domesticated animals today. But ruminant animals, then and now, have special bacteria and protozoa in their digestive tracts that efficiently transform the unsaturated fats and carbohydrates found in plants into saturated fats that compose their bodies' makeup.

It turns out that the amount of saturated fat in ruminant animals such as cattle, deer, sheep, and bison, regardless of whether they are wild or domesticated, varies very little and is irrespective of whether they consume grains or wild grasses. In *Nourishing Traditions,* Sally Fallon explains that buffalo fat is actually more saturated than beef fat and that only 4 percent of the *adipose tissue* of all ruminants is polyunsaturated.

DEFINITION

Adipose tissue is a type of body tissue that contains stored cellular fat, serves as a source of energy, cushions and insulates vital organs, and is active in the formation of hormones.

Furthermore, hunter-gatherer societies hunted animals selectively. They preferred the older male animals because of the abundant insulating fat found along their backs. Among the larger animal species like bison, this slab of fat could weigh 40 pounds or more. Our ancestors also consumed fatty bone marrow, and many used the highly saturated fat of the abdominal cavity to make pemmican and similarly preserved foods. In hunter-gatherer societies, nothing went to waste. The rich, fatty organ meats and the animal's blood were often consumed, and these were considered the most prized delicacies of a kill. Even small game like opossum, beaver, armadillo, and fish provided rich sources of fat in traditional primitive diets.

Benefits of Naturally Saturated Fats

The much-cited Framingham Heart Study, which supports the lipid theory of cardiovascular disease mentioned in Chapter 2, has become synonymous with remarkable advances made in the prevention of heart disease in the United States and throughout the world. Incredibly, the pertinent facts of the Framingham study do not bear this out.

In July 1992, William Castelli, MD, the long-term director of the Framingham study, reported in the *Archives of Internal Medicine* that, "in Framingham, Massachusetts, the more saturated fat one ate, the more cholesterol one ate, the more calories one ate, the lower people's serum cholesterol … we found that the people who ate the most cholesterol, ate the most saturated fat, ate the most calories, weighed the least, and were the most physically active."

Renowned lipid chemist Michael Gurr, PhD, concurs, stating that, whatever might be the cause of coronary heart disease, it cannot be attributed to the intake of saturated fat. In fact, the opposite seems to be the case. According to eminent lipids scientist Mary Enig, PhD, saturated fats are necessary for the proper utilization of the *essential* fatty acids—EFAs are those fats that must be present in our diets—and are necessary for the proper modeling of our bones. Furthermore, she contends that the consumption of saturated fatty acids also results in a reduction of $Lp(a)$ in the blood, and that saturated fats like those found in meats and coconut oil protect the liver from the affects of alcohol ingestion, too.

> **DEFINITION**
>
> **Lp(a),** also called *Lipoprotein(a),* is a subclass of lipoprotein. Numerous genetic and epidemiologic studies have identified Lp(a) as a marker for atherosclerosis, coronary heart disease, and stroke. *Lipoproteins* are particles that transport lipids (fats) and triglycerides around the body in the blood.

No traditional culture in the world has ever been found to be 100 percent vegetarian. There are, however, several cultures—such as the Masai of Africa, some of the Plains Indians, the Inuit, and the Sami—that have traditionally subsisted almost entirely on flesh foods and have been very healthy. Yet when they adopted modern diets, high in refined carbohydrates, the health of these people deteriorated rapidly.

Epidemiological research conducted by Dr. Weston A. Price and corroborated by others shows that it is the introduction of refined carbohydrates in combination with the reduction of traditional saturated fats that results in the people of traditional cultures developing a high incidence of degenerative diseases—especially heart disease.

Since 1957, the publicity given to the hypothesis implicating cholesterol and saturated fats such as coconut oil as the cause of heart disease and cancer has prompted many people to erroneously adopt a totally or mostly vegetarian diet. The author of *Your Body is Your Best Doctor,* H. Leon Abrams Jr., MA, EDS, warns, however, "Whenever eating meat … one would be wise to eat part of the fat, as it is essential to good health. Too often we turn up our noses at the fat and thus waste the part that is of prime importance for balanced nutrition."

The Research of Dr. Weston A. Price

In the early 1930s, Cleveland dentist Weston A. Price embarked on a 10-year journey to investigate how people who had been untouched by modern civilization lived, in order to discover which factors were responsible for excellent dental health. What his investigations revealed was that narrow dental arches, crowding, and cavities were the result of inadequate nutrition.

Price studied people in isolated Swiss villages, the indigenous tribes in the Americas, the Gaelic people of the Outer Hebrides,

Melanesian and Polynesian islanders, African tribes, Aborigines in Australia, and the Maori of New Zealand. Regardless of where his travels took him, Dr. Price found that people who maintained nutrient-rich native diets were remarkably free of disease, had beautifully aligned and decay-free teeth, had fine physiques, and enjoyed exceptional health and vitality.

Upon analyzing the foods these isolated people ate, he discovered that, compared to the American diet of that time, the traditional diets provided more than 4 times the water-soluble vitamins and minerals and 10 times the amount of fat-soluble vitamins! These nutrients were eaten in the form of butter, organ meats, coconut and palm oils, animal fats, and in the eggs of fish and birds that have come to be thought of as unhealthy in modern times.

Yet traditional peoples have instinctively known what scientists of that time had only recently discovered: that fat-soluble vitamins are indispensable because they act as catalysts in the absorption of minerals and in the body's ability to utilize proteins. Without them, we cannot absorb minerals regardless of how abundant they may be in our diets. Through extensive research and careful observation, Dr. Price ultimately discovered a "new" nutrient, which he called *Activator X*. He found that all primitive peoples had a source of Activator X.

DEFINITION

Activator X is vitamin K_2. It was once thought that the benefits of vitamin K were limited to its role in blood clotting, and that vitamins K_1 and K_2 were simply different forms of the same vitamin and possessed the same physiological functions. It is now known that, among other things, the benefits of vitamin K_2 include promotion of bone, cardiovascular, skin, brain, and prostate health.

The isolated groups of people Dr. Price studied also understood the importance of parental nutrition prior to conception. Many of the cultures called for a strict period of special food consumption—high in Activator X content—by both of the potential parents in preparation for the conception of a child. The same nutrient-rich, high-fat foods were considered important for pregnant and lactating women and growing children as well. These foods were particularly rich in minerals as well as in the various fat-soluble activators found only in saturated fats.

According to Dr. Mary Enig, Price was often called to the bedsides of people who were dying. Because of his discovery of the value of Activator X, he would bring with him a bottle of cod liver oil and a bottle of high-vitamin butter oil taken from cows eating fresh grass. Incredibly, when he would place drops of each oil under the tongues of these patients, more often than not the dying person would recover. On the other hand, he noted that when he administered either the cod liver oil or the butter oil alone, he seldom had the same good results. Dr. Enig proposes that the saturated fatty acids in the butter helped the unsaturated fatty acids in the cod liver oil synergistically by simultaneously opening both omega-3 and omega-6 pathways of nutrition for *prostaglandin* production.

> **DEFINITION**
>
> **Prostaglandins** are naturally occurring fatty acids that act as localized hormones. They stimulate contractility of smooth muscle and the uterus. They have the ability to lower blood pressure and to regulate body temperature, blood platelet aggregation, and acid secretion in the stomach. They also control inflammation and vascular permeability and affect the action of certain hormones.

Many traditional dishes provide this sort of synergistic combination of omega-3 and omega-6 saturated fatty acids. Familiar examples include lox and cream cheese, caviar and sour cream, salmon and Béarnaise sauce, and dark-green vegetables cooked in butter. While these factors are found mostly in animal fats, in the traditional Polynesian diet, coconut oil, fish, and/or pork provided the necessary fatty acids. Some Native American cultures found them in a combination of fish or bear fat and evening primrose oil. Traditional combinations of good fats, therefore, should be embraced. Good fats provide factors that open the two critical prostaglandin pathways upon which vibrant health relies.

Studying Other Traditional Societies

There's a mantra that says, "eat fat, get fat—eat lean to stay lean." But there are several examples of traditional cultures that continue to be a consternation to those who would have us avoid fat and cholesterol at all costs. The Inuit people and the Masai and Samburu tribes of Kenya are a few cases in point.

The Inuit people are traditionally arctic hunter-fishermen. They are a cultural group of Canadian Eskimo who subsist on whale, walrus, caribou, seal, and other indigenous creatures. So the typical Inuit diet is high in protein and extremely high in fat. In fact, the Inuit consume from 75 to 90 percent of their calories in the form of fat. Because it is impossible to cultivate crops in arctic conditions, the Inuit only gather and consume the few wild plants that become available during the region's short warm period, which includes a limited variety of grasses, seaweed, roots, and berries.

In the 1920s, anthropologist Vilhjalmur Stefansson studied and lived among a group of Inuit people to discover how the Inuit's extremely low-carbohydrate diet had no adverse effect on their health. Stefansson and his companions spent more than 11 years exploring the arctic and studying its indigenous people. For nine of those years Stefansson, too, lived almost exclusively on meat and enjoyed good health as is recounted in his book, *The Friendly Arctic.* Stefansson proposed that the Inuit were able to get the vitamins and minerals they needed without the addition of any plant-based foods because adequate amounts of vitamin C and other nutrients were present in their diet of raw meats, liver, whale skin, and blubber. The animals they ate had stores of these nutrients in the tissues of their muscles, organs, and fat. Although nutrition experts were extremely skeptical at the time, his conclusions have since been proven valid.

Following their investigations, Stefansson and one of his companion explorers voluntarily agreed to be clinically studied while subsisting exclusively on meat for one year. The results of this rigorous study were reported in a series of articles published in 1930 in the *Journal of Biological Chemistry.*

During the experiment, the men ate beef, lamb, veal, pork, and chicken, which included muscle tissue, liver, kidney, brain, bone marrow, bacon, and fat. The summary and conclusions as reported in the study *Clinical Calorimetry: Prolonged Meat Diets With a Study of Kidney Function and Ketosis* were as follows:

- Stefansson and his colleague, Andersen, lived on an exclusively meat-based diet for one year. The amount of lean meat and fat that was eaten was left up to each of the individuals.

- The daily content of their diets varied from 100 to 140 grams for protein, 200 to 300 grams for fat, and 7 to 12 grams for carbohydrate (from the glycogen in the meat). Total daily caloric intake ranged from 2,000 to 3,100 calories.
- At the end of the one-year experiment, both subjects appeared mentally alert, were physically active, and showed no specific physical changes in any of the body's systems.
- During the first week, both men lost weight due to water loss, which is consistent with initial adjustment to a low-carbohydrate diet. Subsequently, their weights maintained a constant level.
- In the test year, the blood pressure of one man remained constant (105/70); the systolic pressure of the other decreased 20 points and the diastolic pressure remained unchanged (from 140/80 to 120/80).
- Bowel control was not disturbed while the subjects remained on the meat diet. In one instance, when protein calories exceeded 40 percent of daily intake, diarrhea resulted.
- Vitamin deficiencies did not develop.
- Urine acidity during the experiment was two to three times that the acidity resulting from a mixed diet and acetonuria was present throughout the experiment. (Consistent with a low-carbohydrate diet.)
- Urinalyses, blood constituent tests, and kidney function tests showed no evidence of kidney damage.
- While on the diet, the subjects metabolized foods with FA:G ratios between 1.9 and 3.0 and excreted 0.4 to 7.2 grams acetone in their urine per day.
- The clinical observations and laboratory studies showed no evidence of any ill effects had occurred in the men during prolonged exclusively meat diet.

The Samburu people are another group that continues to confound the fat and cholesterol phobic among us. The Samburu have an interesting diet that consists of drinking nothing but milk for three days and then eating nothing but meat for one. Although the routine may vary slightly, generally speaking there are three milk days to every one meat day.

The Samburu's milk is raw and fermented, similar to yogurt, and between their milk and meat the tribesmen consume 400 grams of fat per day! To put this into perspective, the average American with heart disease, obesity, and high blood pressure consumes a mere 80 grams of fat per day.

By tribal tradition, between the ages of 14 and 34, Samburu warriors are not allowed to consume anything but meat and milk and only occasionally a little tree bark tea. No vegetables or fruit are eaten.

Also well documented are the Samburu's neighbors, the Masai. The Masai's traditional diet consists of raw meat, raw milk, and raw blood from their cattle. In the summer of 1935, Dr. Weston A. Price studied the Masai and reported that in Kenya most tribes were completely disease free. The Masai drank an average of seven quarts of very rich whole milk per day, and their diet was approximately 60 percent saturated fat.

Dr. George V. Mann, a Johns Hopkins–educated biochemist and physician, also studied the Masai and Samburu extensively. In his attempt to test the popular assertion that consuming fat and cholesterol increased the risk for heart disease, he looked to the African tribesmen for answers. After having studied 1,500 Masai, he concluded that "they have very low levels of cholesterol in their blood, half as much as we do, and very rarely have cardiovascular disease."

Mann and his colleagues found that both tribes had consistently normal blood pressure and no obesity. Additionally, there was a complete absence of rheumatoid arthritis, osteoarthritis, and gout. He observed that the average tribal child had a cholesterol value of 138; the average American child's was 202 at that time. As tribesmen aged, Mann found that their cholesterol values went down, whereas aging Americans' values went up. Of those people over 55, the mean African cholesterol value was 122, while similarly aged Americans averaged a value of 234.

Dr. Mann contends that a "heart Mafia" has been misinforming the public. "When we find the real cause and prevention of the cholesterol problem, it will seem to many that there was an unwholesome conspiracy."

Chewing the Fat

Another interesting way of examining fats and how they impact health is by looking at how they are used in the livestock feed industry. There once was a time when if you were able to raise a fatter pig than your neighbor, it was considered a good thing. Fat was "in." Lard was a staple food in those days. And obviously, a large pig weighed more than a thin pig, so farmers would make more money if they could sell a heavier animal.

Farmers and ranchers are, by necessity, bright and innovative people, and they discovered long ago that by feeding pigs polyunsaturated fats (in the form of long-chain triglycerides [LCTs] found in oils of soybean and corn) they could create a fatter animal. This is the direct impact of consuming the longer-chain fatty acids found in vegetable oils as opposed to saturated fats, and it is well documented in scientific literature.

Today, however, consumers' demands have made an about-face. Everyone in the supermarket is on the lookout for the best deal on lean meat. People do not want to see a thick ring of saturated fat encircling their pork chops. So how does a modern farmer manage to produce a lean pig?

According to the Department of Animal Science at North Carolina State University, the farmer must stop feeding his pigs polyunsaturated fats and switch them over to saturated fats during their "finishing time" before slaughter. In trials to prove this effect, they initially used beef tallow to finish the pigs, but it was found that tallow was too difficult on the pigs' digestion. The alternative? Switch the pigs to coconut oil, an easily digestible, plant-based saturated fat.

So now we have lean pork. But what are the fats found on the shelves of our supermarkets? For the most part, they are polyunsaturated fats—mostly soybean oil—the same fats that have been historically used to fatten livestock by the animal feed industry. While the saturated fats considered staples in the diets of our ancestors are being fed to livestock in the interest of producing lean animals, we now have lean pigs and obese people.

MCTs' Effects: Energy, Cardiovascular Health, and Aging

It has sometimes been proposed that saturated fats in the diet inhibit the production of prostaglandins, but as noted by Dr. Enig earlier in this chapter, the opposite is true. Saturated fats in the diet increase the body's ability to utilize essential fatty acids.

Lauric acid, as found in mother's milk and coconut oil, improves prostaglandin production. When lauric acid is present in the diet, the long-chain EFAs end up in tissues where they belong, even when EFA content in the diet is relatively low.

Energy and Exercise

One Japanese study conducted by N. Nosaka and colleagues compared the effects of consuming long-chain fatty acids as opposed to the medium-chain triglycerides (MCTs) in coconut oil on the endurance of athletes. Their conclusion stated that consuming a small amount of MCT oil suppresses the rate of perceived exertion (RPE) during moderate-intensity exercise. Furthermore, the data showed a longer duration of subsequent higher-intensity exercise, at levels that exceeded those which were achieved by consuming LCTs.

These days, scandals involving athletes who use illicit performance-enhancing drugs are regularly in the news. Perhaps the news of coconut oil's ability to healthfully enhance athletic performance and increase endurance may save young athletes from the perils of steroids and other dubious synthetic substances.

Interestingly, MCTs provide nearly 10 percent fewer calories than LCTs, too. According to Dr. Ward Dean, a renowned pioneer of innovative nutritional protocols for delaying aging and ameliorating age-related diseases, there are 8.3 calories per gram of MCT oil as opposed to 9 calories per gram of LCTs. That certainly is a unique advantage for calorie counters, but as far as exercise is concerned, what is most important is how rapidly MCTs can be used by the body. MCTs' special structure allows them to be immediately converted into fuel for use by organs and muscles. MCTs are able to cross cells' mitochondrial membranes very rapidly, without a need for the presence of carnitine as LCTs have. This results in the availability of extra amounts of a substance known as *Acetyl coenzyme A*, which ultimately results in the production of ketones.

Scientists attribute the increased energy and endurance that comes from consuming coconut oil to this rapid formation of ketone bodies. Therefore, coconut oil is a good choice for anyone who has increased energy requirements—as when preparing for or recovering from surgery, during periods of rapid growth and development, to enhance athletic performance, and as a work-around for the older population whose normal energy production decreases with age. The MCTs in coconut oil are also becoming popular among bodybuilders and other athletes who adhere to low-carbohydrate diets, as they generally have little or no surplus fat of their own to spare.

Appetite and Weight Control

Fats add a sense of satiety to your eating experience—a satisfying feeling of having had enough to eat. MCTs, in particular, have been shown not only to provide this sense of satiety, but to actually suppress appetite. This is an obviously beneficial advantage for those attempting to lose weight by reducing the number of calories con- sumed. In a 14-day study, six healthy male volunteers were allowed unlimited access to one of three diets: a low MCT diet, a medium MCT diet, and a high MCT diet. Data showed that the total calories consumed by the high MCT diet volunteers were significantly lower than those on the other two diets. The researchers noted that substi- tuting MCTs for other fats in a high-fat diet could prevent the intake of excess energy (in the form of calories) and thereby prevent weight gain in people who consume high-fat or calorie-dense diets.

In addition to the fact that MCTs are more satiating and have a slightly lower caloric value than LCTs, MCTs are not stored in fat deposits in the body. In fact, the MCTs of coconut oil have been shown to enhance *thermogenesis*, which is the burning of fat.

DEFINITION

Thermogenesis is the process of metabolic heat production in warm- blooded animals. As a significant component of the metabolic rate, thermogenesis stimulates an increase in energy expenditure and fat oxidation (that is, fat burning).

So coconut oil offers a triple benefit to weight loss:

- It is lower in calories than other fats.
- It is not readily stored as fat in the body.
- It enhances metabolism to burn even more calories.

This third property may be due to the fact that MCTs in coconut oil behave metabolically in some ways that are similar to carbohydrates (because they are rapidly available for energy), as well as their role in producing ketone bodies as previously mentioned.

As it happens, ketone production is at the foundation of the Atkins low-carbohydrate diet, for example. Consuming MCTs, therefore, should enable people who follow a low-carbohydrate diet to more rapidly obtain weight loss and more easily adhere to the program. Furthermore, ketones are also one of the two substances the brain can utilize for energy (glucose being the other), and they have been found to be the preferred fuel for both the brain and the heart.

Atherosclerosis

Among Filipinos, the Bicolano cuisine is especially noted for its prominent use of chile peppers and coconut milk. Of the 13 regions in the Philippines, Bicol has the highest intake of fat from coconut because nearly all of its food is prepared in coconut milk. And among the Philippine population, Bicolanos have the lowest percentage of death due to heart disease.

One particular study, conducted by the Philippine Coconut Authority (PCA), showed that even among Bicolanos, those who consumed the most coconut oil had the lowest mortality rate from coronary and cardiovascular disease. This study concluded that those who consumed greater quantities of coconut oil had reduced rates of heart disease because of the coconut's mineral content—potassium and magnesium, in particular.

Another study conducted by the University of the Philippines confirmed that the major coconut-consuming countries have lower incidences of high cholesterol and a low prevalence of heart disease. Singling out the people of the Polynesian Pukapuka and Tokelau islands, who derive 35 to 40 percent of their dietary fat from coconut oil, this study showed average serum cholesterol values to be a low 170 milligrams in males and 176 milligrams in females.

Cholesterol by the Numbers

Total Serum Cholesterol	Range
Below 200 mg/dl	Desirable
200–239 mg/dl	Borderline high
240 mg/dl or higher	High

Source: Mayo Clinic, mayoclinic.com/health/cholesterol-levels/CL00001

Immune System Enhancement and Medicine

According to the PCA, coconut's medicinal uses are many and varied. The PCA recommends drinking buko juice (coconut water) for its good balance of potassium chloride, calcium, and magnesium. The balance and combination of these minerals are helpful in the prevention of renal disorders such as kidney stone formation.

The study concluded that drinking the water from just one young coconut daily (approximately two average glasses) could nearly guarantee the prevention of stone formation in the urinary tract. It also suggested that since this treatment utilizes a natural form of medication, the proposed preventative treatment would be virtually complication-free.

Another study, reported in volume 3 of *Advances in Human Nutrition*, to evaluate the immune-enhancing properties of MCTs like those found in coconut oil, injected rats with a serum known to cause severe autoimmune kidney disease. The researchers then added MCTs to the diet of one group of rats. What they noted was a substantial reduction in the pathological changes in the MTC rats' kidneys. From this, they concluded that MCTs could have a positive impact on the sort of autoimmune reactions that are associated with aging.

Brain Function

Neurodegenerative diseases such as Alzheimer's disease and the various dementias are all over the news. It seems that although senility was once a relatively rare thing, these days it has nearly become the rule rather than the exception. There is hardly anyone who isn't directly affected or knows someone who is directly affected by one of these dreaded diseases.

While the exact triggers for the development of progressively impaired brain function are not yet well understood, the brain's need for a constant supply of fuel offers a key. Without continual and adequate nourishment, brain cells become damaged and begin to die. A cascading effect of inflammation ensues, and if prolonged, serious neurodegenerative diseases result.

New research is showing that coconut oil can supply the brain with a profound source of energy—its preferred source—in the form of ketones. This is especially important for people who suffer from diabetes or any neurodegenerative condition such as Alzheimer's, Parkinson's, ALS, or multiple sclerosis because, as will be discussed in greater detail in Chapter 9, all of these disorders appear to have one thing in common: insulin resistance.

Insulin is the hormone that brings glucose into cells where it can be used for fuel. When the brain becomes resistant to the effects of insulin, the tragic result is diabetes of the brain—type 3 diabetes. When brain cells become resistant to insulin, they are unable to take in the glucose they need, they become malnourished, and they begin to die. But the ketones produced by consuming MCTs, like those found in coconut oil, can fuel the brain and other nervous tissues directly without needing insulin to shunt glucose into cells. Ketones completely bypass the need for glucose metabolism.

Ketones are useful in fueling the nervous tissue of premature newborns, they have been shown to help oxygen-deprived brains to recover, and they have been successfully used in the treatment of severe childhood epilepsy. Coconut oil is considered one of the best foods for healthy brain function because, outside of mother's milk, coconut oil is nature's richest source of ketone-producing MCTs.

The Least You Need to Know

- A diet that is high in naturally saturated fat is healthy, providing vital nutrients that are lacking in a low-fat diet. Until recently, high-fat diets were prescribed by physicians as a successful treatment for difficult diseases.

- Polyunsaturated oils like soy and corn oil were once used to fatten livestock. These days, coconut oil is used to produce lean livestock while the polyunsaturated fats fatten people.

- Coconut oil has positive effects on energy, cardiovascular health, appetite, weight control, immunity, and brain function.

How Coconut Oil Stacks Up Against Other Fats

In This Chapter

- Comparing good fats and bad fats
- Using caution: toxins ahead
- Taking the heat
- Nourishing your 100 trillion living cells

Most supermarket shelves offer row upon row of oils from which to choose: various grades of olive oil, canola oil, peanut oil, corn oil, cottonseed oil, safflower oil, sunflower oil …. The list could go on and on, not to mention the other cooking-fat possibilities like butter, bacon fat, margarines, shortenings, and lard. When you survey it all, a health-conscious person starts to feel he or she needs a degree in lipids science to decide which (if any) fats and oils to use. It's enough to make your brain swim.

On one hand, people are told by certain authorities to avoid all fats in order to maintain health. Other factions say that there are "good" fats and "bad" fats and that ne'er the twain should meet—not on your plate at least. Finally, there is a third consensus warning that even the good fats should only be used in certain ways and that some of those fats can become bad if not handled properly.

So which oils should you use? Which ones should you avoid? Which oils are good for cooking, and which oils are best consumed raw? This chapter will help you make sense of this slippery business and give you the information you need to make an informed decision.

Fats to Eat and Fats to Avoid

For the time being, I'll just cut to the chase and discuss which oils should and shouldn't be included in a healthy diet. Further along I will get into the reasons why, so that you can easily determine how each oil should be used on your own.

Fats are primarily "good" or "bad" based on two main criteria. The first consideration is how much and what kind of nutrition a fat provides. The second question is how stable the fat is under various conditions. Generally speaking (although there are exceptions), the following fats are good to eat:

- Coconut oil
- Red palm oil
- Olive oil
- Butter and *ghee* (especially from organically raised, grass-fed beef)

DEFINITION

Ghee is butter that has been clarified by the removal of its milk solids and is used extensively in the cuisines of India and South Asia.

- Oils and fats from wild-caught, cold-water fish and seafood
- Fats and lard from organically raised meat animals
- Flaxseed and a few other seed oils

TO YOUR HEALTH!

Flaxseed and many of the other seed and nut oils are good sources of essential fatty acids, as you will see in the section "Essential Fatty Acids Are … Essential!" later in this chapter. But they must be handled carefully, or they can end up doing more harm than good.

The following are dietary fats that should be avoided:

- Margarine
- Vegetable shortening
- Liquid vegetable oils (soy, canola, corn, etc.)

- Hydrogenated oils (trans-fats in any form)
- Fats from genetically modified (GMO) crops or from the animals that are fed them

Which Oils Are Not Suitable for Cooking?

Anytime a food is cooked it runs the risk of becoming heat damaged. Oils, in particular, must be stable enough to resist chemical changes when heated. Many oils cannot tolerate high temperatures—or even room temperatures—without oxidizing. Oxidized oils are oils that have been heat damaged, and they form free radicals in your body, which is damaging to your health. Furthermore, they can go on to oxidize the good cholesterol in your body and convert it into bad cholesterol.

AW, NUTS!

The manufacture of liquid vegetable oils such as soy, corn, and canola oil requires heat and/or chemical treatment to separate the oil from the other liquid fractions. This is called *fractionation*. This process oxidizes the oil before it even leaves the factory. If manufacturers did not deodorize the oil before selling it, it would smell so rancid you would never buy it!

Polyunsaturated Fatty Acid (PUFA)

When you eat food cooked with polyunsaturated vegetable oil, such as those listed in the fats to avoid, you inadvertently introduce oxidized cholesterol into your system. When PUFAs are heated and exposed to oxygen in the environment, they go rancid. Oxidized, rancid oil should never be consumed. Doing so can lead directly to vascular disease, cancer, and a number of autoimmune disorders.

Toxic Hydrogenated Oils (Trans-Fatty Acids)

Another type of fat that is not suitable for consumption is trans-fat, or hydrogenated fat. Trans-fats are not suitable for eating in any form—cooked or not. These fats are found in margarines, shortenings, and various processed food products. They are manufactured from PUFAs that have been processed in a way (hydrogenated) that makes them solid at room temperature. These oils become plastic-like in the body, and when eaten, they increase your risk of developing a multitude of chronic debilitating diseases such as Alzheimer's disease, breast cancer, and heart disease. But there's more.

It's bad enough that when people consume trans-fats, those fats take the place of healthy, natural fats in the diet, but they also effectively block the uptake of the essential fatty acids that you might otherwise consume. Because of this, the trans-fats end up being deposited in cell membranes where the essential fatty acids should reside. The plastic-like substance literally gums up the normal functioning of the cells and weakens the integrity of cell membranes. Eventually, the body becomes unable to synthesize the enzymes necessary for converting essential fatty acids into the other fatty acids it needs. This results in a deficiency of important fats that your body should be able to manufacture on its own.

Genetically Modified (Engineered) Fats

To make matters worse, most vegetable oils in the United States are made from crops that have been genetically engineered (GE), such as soy and corn. Oils manufactured from GE crops contain even more toxic potential in the form of substances such as *glyphosate* and *Bt toxin* that have been shown to, among other things, kill human kidney cells at very low exposures.

Finally, all liquid vegetable oils are high in omega-6 fats. And while we need both omega-6 and omega-3 fatty acids in our diets, the ratio of omega-6 to omega-3 is important. According to Dr. Elson Haas in his book *Staying Healthy with Nutrition*, the best ratio of dietary omega-6 to omega-3 ranges from 2:1 to 4:1. Since modern diets already include inordinate amounts of omega-6 fats in manufactured foods and very little omega-3 fat, it is easy to exacerbate that ideal ratio by consuming vegetable oils and invite even more degenerative disease.

Put simply, liquid vegetable oils are not suitable for cooking, and hydrogenated vegetable oils are not suitable for consumption in any form. The key to discovering why this is the case is the ratio of naturally saturated fat to polyunsaturated fat in each of the oils.

The Nutrition Profile of Coconut Oil

As you can see in the following table, coconut oil has the greatest percentage of saturated fat combined with the least percentage of polyunsaturated fat. The saturated fat content makes a fat stable and resistant to oxidation and rancidity at high temperatures. Coconut oil can "take the heat" in the kitchen, whereas flaxseed oil has the least percentage of saturated fat and the highest percentage of polyunsaturated fat. It cannot even tolerate average room temperature without becoming rancid.

Comparative Fat Composition of Vegetable Oils

Oil	Monosaturated	Polyunsaturated	Saturated
Coconut	5.8%	1.8%	86.5%
Red palm	37%	9.3%	49.3%
Corn	12.7%	58.7%	24.2%
Peanut	46.2%	32%	16.9%
Soy	23.2%	57.9%	14.4%
Sesame	39.7%	41.7%	14.2%
Olive	77%	8.4%	13.3%
Safflower	12.6%	73.4%	9.6%
Grapeseed	16.1%	69.9%	8.1%
Canola	58.9%	29.6%	7.1%
Flaxseed	22%	74%	4%

If you go down to the third oil, corn oil, you notice that it seems to have a reasonable amount of saturated fat. What makes this oil unsuitable for cooking is its extremely high polyunsaturated fat content. With so much available unsaturated fat, corn oil is readily oxidized. It has plenty of atoms on its molecular structure just begging to bind with oxygen! Nearly 59 percent by volume to be exact.

Only two commercially available edible oils are suitable for use in cooking:

- Coconut oil
- Red palm oil

The reason is their very high percentage ratio of saturated fat to PUFA content. Neither coconut oil nor red palm oil will degrade appreciably under heat, and each one has special nutritive advantages.

Lard, too, would be an option for cooking, except that (incredibly) commercially available lard has been hydrogenated as well! If, however, you have your own source for freshly rendered lard, it is an excellent choice for many high-heat cooking applications. Finally, butter obtained from organically raised, grass-fed beef is an excellent choice for cooking due to its nutrient value and its high percentage of fat saturation.

AW, NUTS!

Q: What does healthy flaxseed oil become when exposed to even moderate heat?

A: Linseed oil.

Q: What is linseed oil?

A: Linseed oil is used in the manufacture of resins and solvents, as a drying oil in impregnators and varnishes for wood-finishing products, as a plasticizer and hardener in putty, as a pigment binder and solvent in oil paints, and in the manufacture of linoleum. *It is not edible!*

Oils Suitable for Consuming Raw

While some of the fats in the "good fats" list at the beginning of this chapter are suitable for use in cooking, some of them should only be eaten raw. Extra-virgin olive oil and flaxseed oil definitely fall into this category. This is because neither oil is highly saturated. Olive oil is primarily a monosaturated fat, and flaxseed oil is highly polyunsaturated. You will recall from earlier in this chapter that polyunsaturated fats and monosaturated fats are vulnerable to oxidation due to their molecular structure.

```
        O   H   H   H
        ‖   |   |   |
  H—O —C —C —C —C —H
            |   |   |
            H   H   H
```
Saturated Fatty Acids = No double bonds

```
    O   H   H   H   H   H   H   H    ↓    H   H   H   H   H   H   H   H
    ‖   |   |   |   |   |   |   |         |   |   |   |   |   |   |   |
H—O —C —C —C —C —C —C —C —C —C = C—C —C —C —C —C —C —C —C —C —C — H
        |   |   |   |   |   |   |   |   |   |   |   |   |   |   |   |
        H   H   H   H   H   H   H   H   H   H   H   H   H   H   H   H
```
Monosaturated Fatty Acids = One double bond

```
    O   H   H   H   H    ↓    H    ↓    H   H   H   H   H   H   H   H
    ‖   |   |   |   |         |         |   |   |   |   |   |   |   |
H—O —C —C —C —C —C —C = C —C —C = C—C —C —C —C —C —C —C —C —C — H
        |   |   |   |   |   |   |   |   |   |   |   |   |   |   |   |
        H   H   H   H   H   H   H   H   H   H   H   H   H   H   H   H
```
Polyunsaturated Fatty Acids = More than one double bond

> *Although many people believe that olive oil is one of the healthiest oils, this is not the case when it comes to cooking. Olive oil is primarily a monounsaturated fat, which means it has one double bond in its fatty acid structure.*

Monosaturated Fats

Besides olive oil, other sources high in monosaturated fat include macadamia nuts (80 percent), avocados (71 percent), and almonds (70 percent). But olive oil is a special case. Because olive oil varies widely by grade and method of manufacture, different olive oil manufacturers list different smoke points for their oils. Some companies list a temperature very close to the smoke point as their maximum limit for safe heating. While these relatively high temperature limits might be correct for avoiding the creation of huge amounts of harmful substances, they are too high to preserve the unique nutrients (especially *polyphenols*) found in high-quality, extra-virgin olive oil. Because of the oxidation of the nourishing substances in olive oil, as well as the potential for *acrylamide* formation, I don't recommend cooking with extra-virgin olive oil.

DEFINITION

Acrylamide is a substance formed in heated oils, and it is known to cause cancer in animals and nerve damage in humans. Industrially, it is used in the manufacture of dyes, plastics, caulking, food packaging, and some adhesives.

Polyphenols are antioxidants found in certain foods that are believed to also affect cell-to-cell signaling, receptor sensitivity, inflammatory enzyme activity, and gene regulation.

For these reasons, olive oil—especially extra-virgin olive oil—should be consumed raw as in salad dressings or drizzled over cooked foods as a flavorful finishing touch. In the same way, other monosaturated fats should be consumed raw in the natural form of fresh fruit, nuts, or nut butters that contain them.

Flaxseed Oil

Flaxseed oil is an exception to the "don't eat polyunsaturated fats" rule, and it has gotten a lot of good press lately. Flaxseed oil is considered a healthy oil because it is an excellent plant source of omega-3 essential fatty acids. But flaxseed and its oil are definitely not for cooking since its fats are so highly unsaturated.

Flaxseed oil even requires particular packaging because light, heat, and oxygen can easily destroy it. Flaxseed products of the highest quality are made using freshly pressed seeds and are bottled in dark glass containers. They are processed at very low temperatures and are not exposed to light, heat, or oxygen. Never buy flaxseed oil that is not refrigerated, and store it immediately in the refrigerator once you have gotten it home.

Essential Fatty Acids Are ... Essential!

Despite what some health authorities would have people believe, our bodies need fat to live and to remain healthy. Especially important are the essential fatty acids (EFAs). Essential means exactly that— essential. In the same way that vitamins are substances people must obtain from food because our bodies are unable to synthesize them, EFAs are also a necessary part of our diets.

As you have seen in the figures illustrating the molecular structures of fat molecules, any fat molecule is made from a chain of carbon atoms bound to hydrogen atoms. At the tail end of the chain (the omega end) is a carbon atom attached to two oxygen atoms. This is what makes the fat an acid. Your body needs to manufacture 20 different fatty acids in all, and it must accomplish this by using only 2 essential fatty acids: omega-6 (linoleic acid) and omega-3 (linolenic acid).

There are only two essential fatty acids known for humans: *alpha-linolenic* acid and *linoleic* acid. But there are other fatty acids that are "conditionally" essential, including *gamma-linolenic* acid, *palmitoleic* acid, and *lauric* acid (as found in coconut oil).

- **Alpha-linolenic acid** is an omega-3 fatty acid found in plants. It is similar to the omega-3 fatty acids in fish oil, called EPA and DHA. Your body can change alpha-linolenic acid into EPA and DHA. Good sources include flaxseed and walnuts.

- **Gamma-linolenic acid (GLA)** is an omega-6 PUFA that must be obtained from food. It plays a crucial role in brain function and normal growth and development, and it helps stimulate skin and hair growth, maintain bone health, regulate metabolism, and maintain the reproductive system. Good sources include plant-based oils such as borage seed oil, evening primrose oil, and black currant seed oil.

- **Linoleic acid** is an unsaturated omega-6 essential fatty acid. It is used in the creation of arachidonic acid, which is conditionally essential for humans. Good sources are grape seed, poppy seed, and hemp seed oils.

- **Palmitoleic acid** is an omega-7, monounsaturated, conditionally essential fatty acid that increases insulin sensitivity and HDL (good) cholesterol and reduces inflammation in the arteries. It also serves to switch on the hormones that tell you when you're full, and it reduces inflammation associated with eczema and other skin conditions. Good sources include certain seafoods and macadamia nut oil.

- **Lauric acid** is essential for the synthesis of monolaurin, which is integral to immune function against pathogens such as unfriendly bacteria, viruses, yeast, fungi, and parasites. Outside of mother's milk, coconut oil is its best source.

Essential Fatty Acid Quiz

Because of the push to reduce fat in our diets, it is likely that EFAs may be the primary nutrient missing from the American diet. EFAs are found in small amounts in quite a variety of fresh foods, especially in certain seeds, nuts, and whole grains. The American diet, however, often contains an excessive amount of *linoleic* acid (omega-6) while being deficient in *linolenic* acid (omega-3). EFA deficiencies are associated with a wide variety of ailments. Mark each box that applies to you:

❑ I experience nosebleeds, bleeding gums, or bruise easily.

❑ My skin is dry and/or flaky.

❑ I have acne or large pores.

❑ I have eczema, psoriasis, or dermatitis.

❑ My nails and hair are dry and brittle.

❑ My hair is excessively oily or dry.

❑ I have been diagnosed with alopecia (hair loss).

❑ I have scaly patches of skin on my face and/or nose.

❑ I have scaly cracks behind my ears or chronically chapped lips.

❑ I experience frequent diarrhea.

❑ My hair has split ends and is unmanageable.

❑ I have tingling in my extremities (arms, legs, hands, feet).

❑ My wounds seem to heal slowly.

❑ It takes me a long time to recover after exertion or exercise.

❑ My eyes feel gritty and dry.

❑ My eyes do not tear.

❑ I have unexplained weight loss or a lack of appetite.

❑ I eat a very low-fat diet.

❑ I am obese or diabetic.

❑ I am asthmatic or have COPD or emphysema.

❑ I suffer from an attention deficit, nervousness, or irritability.

❑ I smoke tobacco or drink alcohol regularly.

❑ I have a history of urinary tract problems and infections.

❑ I eat margarine instead of butter.

❑ I regularly consume refined sugar in beverages and foods.

❑ I take NSAIDs for pain or inflammation: aspirin, naproxen, Motrin, etc.

❑ I have had more than one miscarriage.

❑ I have been diagnosed with dementia, senility, Parkinson's disease, or ALS.

❑ I have been diagnosed with IBS or Crohn's disease.

❑ I take statin drugs to lower or prevent high cholesterol.

❑ I currently use, or have used in the past, cortisone or prednisone prescription drugs or creams.

❑ I suffer from PMS, ovarian cysts (PCOS), or fibrocystic breast disease.

❑ I've been diagnosed with an autoimmune disorder such as rheumatoid arthritis, lupus, or Sjögren's syndrome.

If you have checked seven or more boxes, you may be suffering from an essential fatty acid deficiency. Augmenting your diet with freshly ground flaxseed; wild-caught, cold-water fish (such as salmon); and coconut oil will go a long way toward correcting any essential or conditionally essential fatty acid deficiencies you may have.

Fatty Acids at the Cellular Level

The human body is estimated to have approximately 100 trillion living cells. The health of your body depends on the health of each of those cells. We live and die at a cellular level. If our cells are healthy, our bodies are healthy. If too many cells become sick, malfunction, and die, tissues begin to die. When too much tissue dies, organs fail and die. And ultimately, organ failures are followed by death to the whole organism.

The health of your cell membranes is critically important to the health of cells. Cell membranes impact your rate of aging, the structural integrity of tissues, metabolism, cardiovascular health, your body's ability to deal with inflammation, and its ability to repair wear and tear. Cell membranes are composed mostly of fatty acids that are held together by *phospholipids*.

DEFINITION

A **phospholipid** is a lipid (fat) consisting of a glycerol bound to two fatty acids and a phosphate group.

Phospholipids serve to align the fatty acids of the cell membrane's bilayer. They are responsible for a cell's elasticity and electrical potentials (as in the conduction of nerve impulses), and they allow nutrients to move in and waste products to move out of a cell.

Cell membranes are not just stretchy walls with windows and doors, however. They are active structures that impact activities both inside and outside of the cell. For example, the types of fatty acids in cell membranes determine how well your cells manage inflammation. If you eat too many French fries and potato chips made with polyunsaturated vegetable oils, your cell membranes will become damaged. Good fats are essential for good cell membrane function. Cell membranes that are in good condition also naturally produce hyaluronic acid to help maintain the structure that connects cells together.

Calcium AEP is another important nutrient for supporting cell membrane health—especially for cells that form the myelin sheathing of nerves. Calcium AEP (2-amino ethyl phosphoric acid), too, depends on good fats for its transport. Other good cell membrane nutrients include essential fatty acids like DHA (essential for cardiovascular health and mood) and phosphatidyl serine (PS) for memory and stress tolerance. Fat-soluble antioxidants, too, help protect cell membranes (like the tocotrienols—E vitamins, CoQ10, and lipoic acid).

So now you know that good, stable fats like coconut oil are essential in the diet. They work together with minerals to form what is known as the membrane integrity factor. Good fats make it possible for cells to maintain control of their environment, allowing the entrance of nutrients but not toxic substances and viruses. They maintain and renew the capacitance function of cell membranes that produces the cell's natural electromagnetic field.

Good fats that do not oxidize can combine with essential minerals to form a lipid mineral complex for the transportation of minerals to where they are needed in the body. They provide a cellular patch for tissue repair. Because coconut oil is so stable, it can aid calcium AEP in its unique role in preserving cell membrane function and the reduction of inflammation in the cells of myelin tissue, bone matrix, kidney glomeruli, the lungs' alveoli, the endothelial lining of capillaries, and the arteries of the retina.

The phospholipids-building properties of good fats, like coconut oil, in combination with calcium AEP and phosphatidyl serine create nutrition that offers excellent nerve support. These phospholipids are highly regarded as memory and coordination nutrients and are known to boost stress tolerance as well. They assist in the recovery from the physical toll taken by emotional stressors, and they are fast-acting nutrients for stimulating short-term memory. This is only one of the important ways coconut oil is helpful in the prevention of neurodegenerative diseases in particular, which will be discussed in detail in Chapter 9.

The Least You Need to Know

- Naturally saturated fats such as coconut oil, red palm oil, and butter are an excellent part of a healthy diet.
- Liquid vegetable oils, vegetable shortenings, and margarines should be avoided.
- Hydrogenated trans-fats, oils from genetically modified crops, and heat-damaged fats and oils are toxic.

- Monosaturated fats (like extra-virgin olive oil) and healthy polyunsaturated oils (like flaxseed oil) should be protected from heat and light and should be consumed raw.
- Healthy fats are essential to the health of every one of the 100 trillion living cells in your body.

The Myriad Health Benefits of Coconut Oil

The health claims surrounding coconut oil number in the many hundreds, and new claims are being made and researched every day. But claims are just that—claims. In Part 3 of this book, you will find proof of coconut oil's ability to accomplish exciting cures and prevent disease. You will also discover practical uses and applications for coconut oil in many common ailments and for treating serious, debilitating disease.

Everything from the common cold to HIV, Alzheimer's disease, heart disease, weight loss and management, thyroid function, and healthy skin and hair is covered. Regardless of whether you are nursing a healthy new baby or are concerned about an ailing elder, you will find answers and helpful information in the chapters of Part 3.

Coconut Oil vs. Viruses, Bacteria, and Yeast

Chapter

8

In This Chapter

- Using coconut oil for natural balance and cleansing
- Dissolving lipid envelopes
- Keeping yeast in check
- An alternative to antibiotics

Louis Pasteur, who invented pasteurization, discovered that most infectious diseases are caused by germs and proposed the "germ theory" of disease. Yet, in his later years, he recanted, "I have been wrong. The germ is nothing. The terrain is everything." What Pasteur meant by this is that if the body (the terrain) is in balance, it will not be affected and overcome by pathogenic germs. Where the body's defenses are in place, germs cannot invade and overwhelm.

While medical (allopathic) doctors are concerned with killing pathogens to reduce and alleviate symptoms of infectious disease, and they use various drug and chemical therapies to achieve this, as Pasteur discovered, there is another way. A naturopathic approach works to bring balance to the body so that the body's own defenses provide protection against invaders and are able to rid the body of pathogens that would do it harm.

Coconut oil is an important tool in bringing about the balance the body needs to naturally strengthen its defenses and usher germy invaders out the door. Even when medical interventions may become necessary, coconut oil can help support the healing process that no medicine can accomplish and only the body is able to achieve.

Herxheimer Reactions (a.k.a. "A Cleansing Crisis")

It is interesting that people who are sick will normally describe their illnesses according to the symptoms they are experiencing. For example, people who have a runny nose, cough, and low-grade fever will say, "I have a cold." This is interesting because it's only partially true. If you just "have" a cold, you wouldn't have any symptoms. People only notice that they have a cold when their bodies' defenses have sprung into action. The miserable symptoms that are part and parcel of the common cold are due to an internal war that is raging. Your body is fighting hard to rid you of a virus it has discovered, and you begin to feel the damage that the battle brings. For example:

- Your runny nose helps wash the virus out of your nasal passages.

- Within a few days, the fluid from your nose may thicken and become opaque. Thick mucus in the nasal passages and upper chest develops to trap the germs, so they can be ejected from your body through sneezing and coughing.

- Your fever works by raising your body's temperature to levels that viruses don't easily tolerate. If your temperature is high enough, the heat will destroy the virus.

The symptoms you feel have more to do with healing than with being sick. Similarly, when your body is fighting to rid itself of a serious invader or toxin, your uncomfortable symptoms will increase. Serious "healing crises" or "detox reactions" are also known as *Herxheimer reactions.*

DEFINITION

Herxheimer reactions are phenomena originally observed in the treatment of syphilis that have since been described in many other illnesses. The reaction is seen as a temporary increase in symptoms when antibiotics or other substances cause a die-off in the offending pathogen. This, in turn, causes the release of toxins and other debris that the immune system must reject and remove from the body.

It is important to note that because coconut oil is so powerful in its ability to kill pathogens such as yeast, viruses, bacteria, and fungi, consuming coconut oil in large, regular doses may precipitate an unpleasant Herxheimer reaction—even if you did not realize you were harboring any of these germs.

If you begin using coconut oil and start to feel worse than you did before, you might conclude that your treatment is not working—or is even making matters worse. To the contrary, such reactions are a sign that your body is cleansing itself and is on the road to recovery.

Just as the uncomfortable symptoms of the common cold indicate your body is fighting germs and trying to heal, Herxheimer reactions are the same. They tell you that your immune system is working and that soon things will be better.

If your healing crisis becomes too uncomfortable, however, it is easily managed. By simply reducing the amount of coconut oil you consume while maintaining adequate hydration, you can return to some level of comfort while your body continues to cleanse and heal. Later, when you feel ready, you can increase the dosage of coconut oil again.

Lipid-Encapsulated Viruses

As discussed in earlier chapters, coconut oil works to disable viruses by dissolving their fatty lipid envelopes and by disrupting viruses' ability to replicate themselves. This is particularly helpful in the case of stubborn viruses and in cases where there is no known effective treatment or cure. AIDS and HIV are two cases in point.

HIV and AIDS

Over the years, medicine has found many ways of managing HIV and AIDS but sadly no cure. AIDS is still considered fatal.

Human immunodeficiency virus (HIV) in a lot of ways is like other viruses such as the common cold. There is, however, one important difference. As described earlier in this chapter, the body is able to overcome and get rid of most viruses by employing the immune system. That isn't the case with HIV. The HIV virus is able to disable certain important cells (T-cells) that are vital to our immune response, and our bodies cannot manage to rid themselves of it.

Instead of our T-cells working to fight the infection, HIV takes them over and uses them to replicate more HIV virus. Our killer T-cells are commandeered, turned into HIV factories, and then destroyed.

When enough of these immune cells have been destroyed, people are unable to fight off even the mildest infection, and HIV becomes the deadly *acquired immunodeficiency syndrome* (AIDS). AIDS is the final stage of an HIV infection. People who are diagnosed with AIDS have severely damaged immune systems and are at risk of dying from even the simplest infection.

Several studies have shown, however, that consuming coconut oil is helpful for reducing the viral load of HIV and AIDS patients, and a reduction in the viral load means being ever closer to being well.

There are many stories, too, of miraculous recoveries and remissions. In 1995, Dr. Mary Enig gave a presentation that was reported in India's national newspaper, *The Hindu*. In the article, the staff writer related Dr. Enig's story of how an HIV-positive infant who had been fed formula that was very high in coconut oil content had become HIV-negative.

In an interview published on *Keep Hope Alive* by Mark Konlee, Chris Dafoe related that in 1996 he thought he had little time left to live. Lab tests showed that his HIV viral load was over 600,000, and his CD4 count was down to 10. After having prepared for his funeral, he decided to take one final vacation in the jungles of Surinam.

While there, he ate what the natives he lived with prepared every day—a dish of cooked coconut. At the end of his two-month "vacation," he returned home to Indiana to find that his viral load was completely undetectable. Chris said that he had gained 32 pounds and was feeling great.

Mononucleosis

Mononucleosis, also called *mono,* is a common illness among young people. The viral infection can leave a person feeling tired and weak for many weeks or months, and it is common to relapse after you think it has run its course. While people infected with mononucleosis will eventually recover without the use of medications, recovery requires plenty of rest and loving care.

TROPICAL TIP

Mononucleosis is nicknamed "the kissing disease" because it is easily spread by mouth contact and through the sharing of foods and drinks.

Mono is believed to be caused by the lipid-encapsulated Epstein-Barr virus. Although the symptoms of mononucleosis will eventually go away, the virus that causes it does not. The virus remains in the body and can become reactivated from time to time. During these rebounds it becomes contagious again and can be spread to others.

Because the Epstein-Barr virus has a lipid envelope, it is easily disabled, and its ability to replicate is disrupted by monolaurin synthesized from the lauric acid in coconut oil. Coconut oil may not destroy all of the virus in a body, but it can significantly reduce the viral load to undetectable levels—sometimes quite rapidly.

TO YOUR HEALTH!

An attorney named David tells of how his daughter in college, and some of her classmates, came down with mono. David sent her a supply of monolaurin pills and instructed her to take them. Within nine days, she called David to report that she was well. His daughter's classmates, who did not receive monolaurin, remained sick for weeks, and some were not well by the end of the semester.

Herpes

Eight types of herpes viruses are known to affect humans:

- Herpes simplex 1—Commonly known as oral herpes, which causes fever blisters.
- Herpes simplex 2—A sexually transmittable disease, genital herpes.
- Varicella zoster—Causes chicken pox and shingles.
- Epstein-Barr virus—Causes mononucleosis, a.k.a. "the kissing disease."

- Cytomegolo virus—A virus that is transmittable from a woman to her unborn child.
- Roseolovirus—Known as 6th disease, roseola infantum, or simply roseola.
- HHV7—Similar to roseolovirus.
- Rhadinovirus—Known as the Kaposi's sarcoma–associated herpesvirus.

While each of these herpes viruses causes different symptoms depending on the system it affects, they all have one common attribute—they all have lipid envelopes that are destroyed by monolaurin. Lauric acid in coconut oil contributes to the synthesis of monolaurin in the body and works to reduce the body's total viral load while the viruses are active—and even after these diseases have run their course and are relatively dormant in the body.

In the case of chicken pox and shingles, I have personally seen that consuming coconut oil can reduce the relative proliferation of lesions. Topical application of coconut oil to the affected areas of the body reduces or completely prevents scarring, too.

Measles

The measles virus is highly contagious and can be deadly. It is transmitted from person to person by droplets that are sprayed from the infected person when he or she sneezes or coughs. The measles virus can even remain in the air to infect others for up to two hours after an infected person has left a room.

Measles is a *paramyxovirus*—a group of RNA (ribonucleic acid) viruses that are predominantly responsible for acute respiratory diseases. They are able to enter target cells by fusing their lipid capsules to human cells, thereby gaining entry into the cell's cytoplasm.

Coconut oil in the diet is a good preventative to viruses such as these since coconut oil helps the body maintain healthy cell membranes that allow nutrients in and keep invaders out. It also acts to reduce the impact of measles by dissolving the virus's lipid coating.

Interesting research points to the fact that measles may be responsible for more than a rash and a respiratory infection, however. Measles, as a low-grade chronic intestinal infection, has been implicated as a cause of Crohn's disease, IBS, and other bowel disorders as well. Perhaps this is another reason why Crohn's and IBS patients find relief in coconut macaroons and eating coconut oil. Coconut oil has anti-inflammatory properties to ease intestinal inflammation while being able to deactivate viruses, too.

Hepatitis C

Hepatitis C is a contagious liver disease that results from infection with the hepatitis C virus. It can be a relatively mild illness, or it can become serious, chronic, and life threatening. Most cases of hepatitis C are spread from person to person through blood contact, such as when an infected IV drug user shares a dirty hypodermic needle with someone else. Before 1992 and modern screening practices, hepatitis C was also accidentally spread through blood transfusions and organ transplants.

As far as coconut oil is concerned, inactivating the hepatitis C virus is just another day's work, as it deactivates hepatitis C in the same way it does other viruses. It dissolves its fatty lipid envelope. But because hepatitis C does its damage in the liver, coconut oil plays a second important role.

Viruses and free radicals can do incredible damage to the liver, but coconut oil works to protect the liver from both possibilities. Coconut oil contains a high concentration of healthy medium-chain fatty acids that support liver health. When ingested, these medium-chain fatty acids travel directly to the liver and immediately begin helping the immune system fight infection. Because coconut oil is so stable, it acts as an antioxidant in the liver, disarming free radicals and inhibiting the formation of new ones. If that were not enough, medium-chain fatty acids support the liver in regenerating tissue when the liver has been damaged.

Influenza and the Common Cold

Coconut oil has even been shown to work its magic on dangerous
SARS and influenza viruses. According to the Centers for Disease
Control, over the period of 30 years between 1976 and 2006, deaths
associated with the seasonal flu in the United States ranged from a
low of about 3,000 to a high of about 49,000 people. Some people,
such as the elderly, the very young, pregnant women, and people
with compromised immunity, are at an increased risk for serious flu
complications and death. Routine consumption of coconut oil can
be especially helpful to those at high risk for complications, and it
can be an aid in getting them through the virus if and when it is
contracted.

A cold virus, on the other hand, is not nearly so dangerous. Yet the
symptoms of a flu infection and the common cold are often confused
because they generally begin in the same manner—coughing, sore
throat, achiness, and a general feeling of being unwell. Because of
this, you might be thinking that coconut oil could swiftly dispatch a
cold, too. What a boon that would be! But the viruses that cause the
flu are not like the rhinovirus that causes a cold. Cold viruses are not
lipid encapsulated, so coconut oil cannot disable them in the same
way it does so many other viral invaders. Coconut oil may still be
very useful during a bout with a cold, however.

At any given moment there are potentially millions of pathogens
bombarding our immune system, and a great number of these are
vulnerable to the effects of consuming coconut oil. When we acquire
a miserable infection like a cold, our poor immune systems are
working double-time. Our bodies are working hard to rid us of that
virus, but also to rid us of less obvious pathogens as well. Consuming
coconut oil during a bout of the common cold relieves the immune
system from having to work so hard. Coconut oil disables the
viruses, yeast, and bacteria that are vulnerable to medium-chain fatty
acids, while the immune system can mostly concentrate on getting
you past your cold.

Yeast (*Candida albicans*)

Candidiasis is an infection caused by an overgrowth of yeast. There are more than 20 species of Candida, but the species that causes people the most trouble is *Candida albicans*. These organisms live everywhere. They thrive happily in our digestive tract and even on the surface of our skin—usually causing no problems. But when the conditions are right, candida can have a population explosion and cause infection. The widespread use of broad-spectrum antibiotics is often the cause. See Chapter 1 to discover whether you have many risk factors for a candida infection.

Antibiotics are used to kill infectious bacteria. Unfortunately, they kill lots of good bacteria at the same time. When lots of bacteria die off, their absence leaves room for candida to expand and take over. Typical candida infections include vaginal yeast infections, oral thrush, diaper rash, and infections of the nail bed. But candida can do more than that. It can cause a systemic infection, too. A systemic yeast infection is a serious condition that may not be easily recognized. Symptoms include the following:

- In anyone: Headache, fatigue, brain fog, digestive problems, allergies, depression, poor memory, and general irritability.

- In children: Restlessness, poor performance in school, hyperactivity, chronic ear infections (otitis media), and stomachache.

- In women: Recurrent vaginal yeast infections and recurrent bladder infections.

- In men: Recurrent jock itch, persistent athlete's foot fungus, impotence, and prostatitis.

The capric and caprylic acids in coconut oil can stem the tide, however. These medium-chain fatty acids have powerful antifungal properties. Applied to the skin, coconut oil will reduce the inflammation and discomfort of a yeast infection while it kills the yeast. Taken internally, coconut oil will sweep the digestive tract of the marauders and prevent them from spreading to other organs via your blood. Made into a refrigerated suppository, it brings instant comfort to a vaginal or anal inflammation.

Bacteria

Most bacteria are harmless. Some, in fact, are actually quite helpful, even necessary, for our survival. *Lactobacillus acidophilus* bacteria, for instance, live in our intestine and help us digest food, provide nutrients, destroy disease-causing microbes, prevent yeast overgrowth, and even fight cancer cells. Less than 1 percent of bacteria cause disease in people. But if a bad bacterium gains a foothold or a good bacterium ends up in the wrong place, it can multiply and cause problems.

Helicobacter pylori

Helicobacter pylori (H. pylori) bacteria infect the stomach lining. H. pylori is usually acquired during childhood, and approximately 50 percent of people harbor it. Most people never have any symptoms of an H. pylori infection, though. If, however, you develop a peptic (stomach) ulcer, you probably have H. pylori to thank. Dr. Bruce Fife says that 90 percent of all stomach ulcers are due to an H. pylori infection.

Unlike in the case of viral and yeast infections, antibiotics can be used to treat bacterial infections like those caused by H. pylori. But there is a drawback to that approach. When antibiotic therapy is used, many of the good bacteria die along with the bad. As previously mentioned, when this happens it opens the door to yeast overgrowth. Furthermore, bacteria of all kinds are becoming dangerously resistant to drug therapies. Eventually, we will run out of antibiotic options at a time when bacteria will be more formidable than ever before.

The medium-chain fatty acids in coconut oil are able to kill H. pylori and other bacteria without triggering resistance in them. In fact, using coconut and coconut oil regularly may prevent infection altogether while allowing the friendly bacteria to thrive and hold yeast populations in check.

Cystitis

Cystitis is a urinary tract infection (UTI) that is usually caused by bacteria such as *Escherichia coli* (E. coli). These bacteria enter through the urethra and infect the bladder. Left unchecked, they can migrate to the kidneys and cause infection there, too.

Women are more prone to cystitis than men because their urethra is in close proximity to the anus. Additionally, pressure from pregnancies and traumas from childbirth may make the bladder less likely to empty completely so bacteria are never completely flushed out. Anyone who suffers from recurrent UTIs will be happy to know that much research shows that coconut oil may be useful in the treatment of bladder and kidney infections.

One particular study induced kidney failure in rats. In this study, rats who were fed coconut oil developed fewer kidney lesions, and the ones they did develop were less severe, demonstrating that coconut oil has a protective effect on the urinary tract.

In *The Coconut Oil Miracle*, Dr. Fife writes about a woman who consulted him for a bladder infection. After he told her about the antibacterial properties of coconut oil, the woman decided to begin taking it immediately in hopes of resolving the problem. It turned out that, without any other treatment, the bladder infection was gone in just two days. Dr. Fife says he was so impressed that he has begun recommending coconut oil routinely for bladder infections and that he is seeing good results. For people who are plagued with recurrent bladder infections, it is "the coconut oil miracle" indeed!

The Least You Need to Know

- Coconut oil is a powerful internal cleanser. It can augment the actions of the immune system by killing pathogens in the body. Sometimes these die-offs can make you feel worse for a time, but that is a sign of healing.
- Coconut oil is highly effective at killing off lipid-encapsulated viruses such as those responsible for herpes, mono, measles, and hepatitis C.

- Yeast overgrowth can be prevented and corrected by regularly using coconut oil in the diet and on the skin.
- Commonly bothersome bacteria like E. coli and H. pylori are destroyed by coconut oil without triggering the bacteria to mutate into more dangerous, drug-resistant forms.

Dementias and Neuropathologies

In This Chapter

- The coconut oil "cure"
- The structures behind the symptoms
- Drugs that harm, ketones that nourish
- Coconut oil: the caregiver's friend

Alzheimer's dementia (AD) is the world's most frequently diagnosed form of dementia, accounting for up to 70 percent of all diagnoses. After Alzheimer's dementia, the second-most-diagnosed dementia is Lewy body dementia, which accounts for up to 20 percent of all dementia cases. In fact, more than 35 million U.S. elders have been diagnosed with dementia of one type or another, and the numbers are growing at an incredible rate of one new case every 7 seconds worldwide! The tragedy of dementia, however, is only one facet of neurodegenerative disease.

Other neurodegenerative diseases that are growing in prevalence include amyotrophic lateral sclerosis (ALS, also called Lou Gehrig's disease), Parkinson's disease (PD), multiple sclerosis (MS), Huntington's disease, vascular dementia, and frontotemporal lobe dementia. Even as long as it is, this is not an exhaustive list.

Every day these dreaded disorders steal people's precious memories. They rob loved ones of their independence. They wipe out dreams of future achievements and erase the possibility of creating new plans and goals. The ability to reason evaporates, and people are left mere shadows of the richly integrated and dynamic beings their families have known and loved. But now, for the first time since this avalanche of disorders began to descend, there appears to be real hope on the horizon. This chapter explores the exciting possibilities of how coconut oil fits into some likely answers.

Purported Benefits

News flash: *Coconut oil may stop, reverse, or even cure Alzheimer's disease!* Now, if you have been reading along since the first chapter, you will recall that "there is no such thing as a panacea." If, however, coconut oil can reverse or even cure Alzheimer's disease, what can't it do? Maybe there is a panacea after all.

In her fascinating book *Alzheimer's Disease: What if There Was a Cure?*, Mary Newport, MD, describes her husband's journey through AD and the reprieve they discovered in the form of coconut oil. It turns out that the medium-chain triglycerides (MCTs) in coconut oil are converted by the liver into ketones, which are the brain's preferred fuel.

According to Dr. Bruce Fife and others, recent discoveries have shown that the brains of dementia patients are insulin resistant. They have a form of diabetes of the brain—diabetes type 3. Insulin resistance makes it difficult or impossible for tissues to use glucose (sugar) as fuel, and without fuel brain tissue will die. Ketone bodies that are formed when coconut oil is consumed provide an alternative fuel for the brain and other affected nervous tissues.

Once placed on ketone therapy, typically in the form of a ketogenic diet (described in Chapter 11) augmented by the consumption of MCT oils, many patients experience improved memory and cognition, the ability to resume favored activities, a return of personality, and the ability to interact socially. These sorts of results are barely short of miraculous.

A Little Bit of Brain Science

To appreciate the beauty of how MCTs work in stalling or reversing the symptoms of neurodegenerative diseases, it is necessary to know a little bit about the brain and other nervous tissues. There are three main structures of the human brain: the *brain stem*, the *cerebellum*, and the *cerebrum*. Each area within these structures serves to facilitate or control a complex set of functions, some of which are duties shared with other areas.

- The **brain stem** is at the uppermost position of the spinal cord, and its duties are among the most primitive functions of the brain. It regulates involuntary actions such as breathing, heart rate, and to some extent digestion.

- Located at the upper-rear of the brain stem, below and behind the cerebrum, is the **cerebellum**—the brain's center for posture, balance, and movement.

- The **cerebrum** is the largest of the three main brain structures and occupies the uppermost space in the skull's cranial cavity. Its duties include the higher-order functions. Its left *cerebral hemisphere* is primarily responsible for producing and understanding speech, mathematics, reading, and writing. Damage to the left hemisphere often results in problems with verbal communication and with movement on the right side of the body. The right cerebral hemisphere is primarily responsible for visuospatial skills, an appreciation of art and music, a sense of physical direction, attention, and the regulation of emotions. Damage to the right cerebral hemisphere will often affect movement on the left side of the body and visuospatial abilities. The injury or death of brain cells, whether incurred from toxins, a stroke, or a disease process, affects a person's ability to function according to where in the brain the injury occurs.

DEFINITION

A **cerebral hemisphere** is one of the halves of the cerebrum. The left and right cerebral hemispheres are divided by a deep fissure and are connected at the base by the corpus callosum. The hemispheres are made up of an external gray layer (the cerebral cortex) and an internal white matter that surrounds gray matter called nuclei (the basal ganglia).

In the dementias, it is often the gray matter of the cerebral cortex and the structures deep in the cerebrum that are primarily involved. The gray matter, or cerebral cortex of the cerebrum, is where thinking, remembering, and reasoning go on. This area of the brain is also responsible for impulses that control a wide variety of muscular activity. In the deepest area of the cerebrum lie the structures of the limbic system, which are responsible for memories, emotions, and learning.

The various progressive dementias and neurodegenerative diseases are differentiated by the areas of the brain and nervous tissues that are involved and, therefore, the resulting symptoms that are present.

Brain Structures in Neurodegenerative Disease States

Structure	Controls	Disease
Cerebral cortex	Voluntary muscle movement	ALS
Basal ganglia	Voluntary movement	Parkinson's, Huntington's
Myelin sheaths	Nerve insulation, conduction	MS
Hippocampus	Short-term memory, thought	Alzheimer's
Frontal lobes	Personality, behavior, language	Pick's

However correct, this explanation is quite an oversimplification. There are many overlaps among the dementias and neurodegenerative disease states. For instance, someone with Lewy body dementia will likely develop Parkinson's disease as well—but maybe not the other way around. A person with Alzheimer's disease may at the same time suffer from vascular dementia or Parkinson's disease. The cells of the brain are so interrelated that rarely do these disorders follow a strict definition.

The Hippocampus

Alzheimer's disease is especially known for the symptom of short-term memory loss. The formation of memory is the domain of the hippocampus, which lies deep within the cerebrum and consists of two "horns" that curve backward from the amygdala. The hippocampus has the important role of converting short-term thoughts and experiences into things you will remember over time—long-term memory.

If the hippocampus is damaged by injury or disease, a person cannot build new memories. Instead, the world becomes a strange place where every experience rapidly fades into oblivion. While older memories from the time before the initial damage are usually left untouched, in the case of progressive dementias, even the older memories eventually fade into obscurity and confusion.

The Hypothalamus

The hypothalamus is integral to emotion and also plays a role in memory. In Lewy body dementia, the aggregate of proteins that are responsible for the disease and damage in the brain collect in the hypothalamus in large proportions. Not only does this affect the ability to remember, but it has the propensity of changing memories and even creating memories of experiences that never occurred—but which are nonetheless very real to the person experiencing them.

In dementias that heavily impact the hypothalamus, people experience unwelcome intrusive thoughts, images, and unpleasant ideas that may become obsessions. These experiences are distressing and can be difficult to be free of and manage. Full-blown delusions and multimodal hallucinations are common and might best be described as something like a cross between post-traumatic stress disorder (PTSD) and schizophrenia.

Drugs—A Help or Hindrance?

With such distressing symptoms, people become understandably desperate for a cure or at least a way to manage all of the difficulties. So far, medical science has no cures, but it does offer many possible "helps" in the form of pharmaceutical drugs.

TO YOUR HEALTH!

All Medicines Are Poison! Dr. Melvin H. Kirschner chose the title for his book as he recalled his first pharmacology lecture in medical school. The professor had pronounced, "Ladies and gentlemen, I am here to teach you how to poison people … [long pause] … without killing them, of course."

Medicines are, of course, potential poisons. Otherwise we would not need doctors to prescribe medications or pharmacists to dispense them. There would be no U.S. Food and Drug Administration to oversee drug trials, approve their use, and monitor their production. There would be no "controlled substances."

The key to whether a medicinal "poison" kills a person, makes him ill, or simply eradicates bacteria lies in the size of the dosage, its frequency, and its duration. Moreover, the patient's physical condition, mental state, weight, age, stage of development, history, metabolism, other medications, and a long list of other variables must be taken into consideration as well.

Considering the complexities of neurodegenerative diseases, the relatively advanced ages of the affected population, the number and types of drugs many elders are already taking, and the sorts of drugs that are available for managing dementias, prescription drugs become a dicey proposition for the elderly.

Statins

Statins, as a rule, are not used to treat dementia or other neurodegenerative diseases. They are, however, widely prescribed to all sectors of the population (even to children) in the interest of lowering cholesterol. In some cases, statins are prescribed as a preventative against developing high cholesterol. Familiar statin drugs include Lipitor, Crestor, Pravachol, Zocor, Mevacor, and Baycol.

The adverse side effects of these drugs are many, including mental deterioration, brain damage leading to memory loss, mood swings, behavioral changes, liver and kidney failure, muscle wasting, and death. Yet somehow, a deeply entrenched fear of cholesterol has managed to make such serious risks acceptable.

In case you have read this far and have not yet picked up on the fact: *Cholesterol is not "the enemy."* Humans absolutely need cholesterol. Our bodies *make* cholesterol. The cells of our body are encased in a lipid membrane composed of fat and cholesterol. Even the membranes of the organelles inside each of our cells are made up of cholesterol.

Cholesterol is a major contributor to all the processes of building, maintenance, and repair our bodies engage in:

- It is essential for proper immune function.
- It is necessary for building strong bones, and it protects against osteoporosis.
- It is an important structural component of every cell— especially nerve cells.
- It is absolutely essential to the brain and for the transmission of nerve impulses and nerve cell communication.

While the brain accounts for only 2 percent of a body's mass, it contains a whopping 25 percent of the body's cholesterol. It's so important that the brain even manufactures its own cholesterol to augment that which is produced in the liver.

That being said, statin drugs, which are designed specifically for reducing serum cholesterol, should be viewed very critically when considering brain health. They effectively reduce the amount of precious cholesterol available to the brain and nervous tissues. Many patients who never experienced problems before report severe mental decline when they begin statin therapy—and sometimes it is irreversible.

Acetylcholine and Cholinesterase Inhibitors

Cholinesterase inhibitors are a class of drugs designed to improve mental function in the demented. Some time ago, scientists noted that some (anticholinergic) medications blocked the neurotransmitter acetylcholine, resulting in brain dysfunctions associated with dementia. From this idea, they proposed that drugs that would inhibit the breakdown of acetylcholine might have the opposite effect and improve brain function.

This is how the common dementia medications such as Exelon (rivastigmine), Aricept (donepezil), and others came about. Ironically, it turns out that many of the same drugs used to treat dementia can actually speed up its progression. And sometimes their side effects are even worse than the diseases they were designed to treat. In fact, in one study, 322 patients were given Aricept while 326 were given a placebo. At the end of just 24 weeks, the Aricept group sustained 11 deaths while the placebo group had none.

Anticholinergic Drugs

Even more ironic than anticholinesterase inhibitors' propensity to aggravate the problems they were designed to treat is the fact that doctors often prescribe them along with *anticholinergic* drugs. The effects of these two classes of drugs work in diametric opposition to one another.

Each cancels out the effects of the other, effectively destroying any good value either one of them may have had. This cancellation effect, however, does not make them innocuous drugs. Both drug types continue to disrupt brain chemistry and produce undesirable side effects as a result.

There is a long list of anticholinergic drugs that elders should avoid because of how they alter brain chemistry. The list includes general anesthetics; psychoactive drugs like Valium, Xanax, Zoloft, Haldol, and Risperdal; antihistamines like Benadryl and Dimetapp; antacids like Pepcid, Zantac, and Tagamet; hypnotics like Ambien, Lunesta, and Sominex; and *NSAIDs* like Vioxx, Advil, Aleve, and Celebrex.

DEFINITION

NSAID is an acronym for nonsteroidal anti-inflammatory drug. These are typically used in place of aspirin or corticosteroids to reduce inflammation, pain, and fever. Their generic names include ibuprophen, naproxen, and celecoxib.

People who suffer from dementia find their symptoms are exacerbated by these drugs, and many healthy people report their first dementia-like episodes after having taken such medications. These drugs have a powerful influence on brain chemistry. In fact, it has been reported that frequent users of Zantac and similar antacids more than double their risk of developing dementia.

It has been long known in the medical community that elders do not metabolize medications in the same way that younger people do. Often a very small drug dosage, one that would be more appropriate for a child, is better suited to an elder than what would normally be prescribed for an adult. In fact, "normal" doses of many medications result in an effect that is exactly opposite of that which was hoped for. Yet our elders are some of the most highly medicated members of society.

Medicating the elderly is always a serious issue, but anticholinergic drugs are a special case. This class of drugs is so powerful that they are prescribed in the treatment of the following:

- Cold and allergy symptoms
- High blood pressure
- Stomach ulcers
- Muscle spasms
- Urinary incontinence and overactive bladder
- Acid reflux (GERD) and heartburn
- Diverticulitis and ulcerative colitis
- Motion sickness
- Asthma and chronic bronchitis
- Parkinson's disease
- Prostatitis
- Urinary tract infections

Obviously, any class of drugs that can affect changes in so many systems of the body is powerful indeed. That means they produce powerful side effects in the elderly as well, including anxiety, delirium, disorientation, confusion, dizziness, memory loss, hallucinations, involuntary muscle twitching, agitation, incoherent speech, seizure, and coma.

The Critical Role of Ketones

While manufactured drugs carry the potential for dangerous side effects, ketones have been used safely for many years in medicine. They have been used therapeutically in the care of premature infants to provide them with the easily metabolized energy they desperately need. Ketones have been used in the care of the malnourished and in people who have difficulty absorbing nutrients from their diets. Athletes use ketones to improve endurance and performance. Weight watchers use ketones to stimulate fat loss while simultaneously reducing appetite. Ketone therapy has even been used in the treatment and cure of epilepsy for over 90 years. Ketones are, in fact, epilepsy's only known cure. Ketones work to bring about homeostasis in the brain and nervous tissues, balancing and normalizing their function. Ketones are like a super-fuel for the brain.

Neurodegenerative diseases are not caused by an inadequate supply of any drug in the diet any more than a toothache is caused by not consuming enough aspirin. We know that the root cause of dementias and neurodegeneration is an inadequate supply of fuel to nervous tissues. If these tissues are wasting away because they cannot use glucose due to insulin resistance, it makes sense to feed the brain with a food it can use—its preferred fuel—ketones.

How Much Coconut Oil to Use

There are a variety of valid suggestions regarding how much coconut oil to include in the diet, ranging from 2 tablespoons per day to 6 or more. Ideally, as much coconut oil as can be tolerated should be consumed—especially if you cannot keep your loved one on a ketogenic diet (described in Chapter 11). Realistically speaking, however, the goal is to start with only 1 or 2 tablespoons per day and gradually increase the dosage, spread over two to four meals.

If you take too much coconut oil too abruptly, it could result in indigestion, diarrhea, or cramping because most people are not accustomed to consuming so much fat. To avoid these symptoms, begin slowly and increase the amount over the course of a week or more. If unpleasant symptoms develop, drop back to a level that had been comfortable for a few days before attempting to increase the dosage again.

In her book *Alzheimer's Disease: What if There Was a Cure?*, Dr. Mary Newport describes how her husband, Steve, experienced a remarkable improvement in mental clarity on his first day of coconut oil therapy, after having eaten only 2 tablespoons of coconut oil in his oatmeal. After long experimentation combined with journaling and charting his results, they have settled on the following routine:

- One 3-tablespoon mixture of 1 part coconut oil and 1 part MCT oil (see Appendix B) at each meal—6 tablespoons in all.
- He eats a low-carbohydrate, whole-foods diet.
- Additionally, he receives a tablespoon each of cod liver oil and fish oil, along with vitamin supplements daily.

How to Fit Coconut Oil into an Elder's Diet

The most successful way I have found to incorporate coconut oil into an elder's diet is by serving familiar foods while substituting coconut oil for the usual fat component. For instance, I might use coconut oil instead of butter on toast, or on baked potatoes or pasta. Or I might add it to the cooking water of dried beans, rice or grits. Another way to add substantial amounts (1 or 2 tablespoons at a time) is to stir it into hot oatmeal (see Chapter 17) or add it to hot cocoa or smoothies.

Coconut oil easily mixes into hot liquids like soups, chili, and sauces, but it tends to solidify when added to cold foods or when refrigerated. This latter effect can be desirable, especially when making candy-like preparations and parfaits. Refrigerated salad dressings that have been made with coconut oil should be warmed and shaken well before serving.

Common Coconut Oil Conversions

When thinking of adding coconut oil to your loved one's diet, be sure to consider all of the other coconut products, too (see Chapter 3). Each of the following contains approximately 1 tablespoon of coconut oil:

- $4^{1}/_{2}$ tablespoons undiluted coconut milk
- One $2\times2\times^{1}/_{2}$-inch piece coconut meat
- 2 tablespoons coconut cream concentrate
- $^{1}/_{3}$ cup grated coconut
- Fourteen 1-gram capsules coconut oil

Dementia Patients Crave Sweets

It's true that, almost universally, dementia patients have an inordinate craving for sweets—way out of proportion to anything most
people are able to imagine. Although this has remained an enigma
to caregivers for many years, we finally have an answer to why this is
so.

Because dementia patients are suffering from chronic low–blood
sugar in the tissues of their brains, the body sends signals telling
them to consume more sweets. But no amount of sugar will ever be
enough to satisfy these cravings because their brains have become
insulin resistant. For all of the sweet foods they consume, little or
none of the glucose in their bloodstreams will ever enter the brain
tissue. The dementia patient's brain is starving.

But this is a wonderful advantage for caregivers who know about
the MCT benefits of adding coconut oil to their loved ones' diets.
When coconut oil is added to desserts and other favorite sweet foods,
the dementia patient will happily consume sufficient quantities of
coconut oil to be of some benefit. When sufficient quantities of
ketones are available to tissues for use as fuel, the hunger and cravings subside.

Eventually, caregivers can gradually move the diet ever closer to a
fully ketogenic diet without the patient enduring painful sugar cravings. Finally, when the ketogenic diet along with additional dosing of
MCT oils has been fully established, the patient will be generating
and consuming an optimal amount of ketones for his or her nervous
system's needs—without further exacerbating the already established
insulin resistance in the brain.

Patients Need Help Absorbing Nutrients

As people age, their ability to absorb nutrients from food decreases appreciably over time. Some of this is due to a reduction in the production of hydrochloric acid that breaks down proteins in the stomach. Other problems result when enzymes from fresh raw foods are not included in great enough quantity in the diet. Older people tend to eat less than their younger counterparts as well. These facts, along with the interference of many over-the-counter and prescription drugs, work together to cause problems of malnutrition due to malabsorption.

Our bodies need sufficient quantities of the macronutrients for optimal health—good fats, proteins, and carbohydrates, along with the vitamins and minerals they contain. To make the best use of the fat-soluble vitamins (A, D, E, and K) and minerals, however, fat is doubly important. Unfortunately, fat has generally been relegated to the "no-go zone" in many nutrition circles. People have become fat deficient, and the fats that they do consume are mostly manufactured polyunsaturated and hydrogenated fats that often do more harm than good.

TO YOUR HEALTH!

The September 2004 issue of *Clinical Biochemistry* reported, "The medium-chain fats in coconut oil are considered so nutritious that they are used in baby formulas, in hospitals to feed the critically ill, those on tube feeding, and those with digestive problems. Coconut oil has even been used successfully by doctors in treating aluminum poisoning."

Coconut oil is an important adjunct to the diets of the elderly principally because it assists the body in its mission to assimilate the fat-soluble vitamins, provitamins, and minerals that are available in foods. If there are tons of vitamins available in our food but no mechanism to access them and take them to the tissues where they are needed, it would be just as if they were not in our food supply at all. This is sad but true, and it is exactly the case with many in the elder population. They eat and eat but do not put on weight. They eat nourishing food but somehow come down with deficiency diseases. They suffer osteomalacia, osteoporosis, goiter, night blindness, macular degeneration and retinopathies, anemia, and even scurvy!

As described in Chapter 6, coconut oil provides one leg of the Activator X factor discovered by Dr. Weston A. Price. It enhances uptake of fat-soluble vitamins. It is especially helpful in vitamin D synthesis (see Chapter 12), a vitamin that is deficient in most elderly. It also acts as a mineral superhighway for transporting vital mineral nutrients to where they are needed for maintaining heart health, teeth and bone mineralization, and healthy cell function.

Special Topical Applications

Straight coconut oil is a wonderful tool for caregivers of the demented. As described in detail in Chapter 12, coconut oil is especially nourishing to the skin and hair. While coconut oil in the diet helps to maintain the health and integrity of skin and hair, topical applications of coconut oil are very helpful, too. Everyone can benefit from coconut oil's moisturizing properties and protection against infection, but the elderly and demented really need the extra care and attention coconut oil provides.

Topical applications of coconut oil and coconut oil–based products help prevent and resolve a number of problems to which dementia patients are prone. Among them are skin tears, rashes and yeast infections, bacterial infections, pressure wounds, and cracked, inflamed, and peeling skin.

"Neat" Applications (Straight Coconut Oil)

Coconut oil is nourishing to the skin and provides a powerful remedy for viruses, yeast, and bacteria that would do harm to fragile and moist areas of skin tissue. Dementia patients however, develop skin problems and other issues that go far beyond run-of-the-mill maintenance and repair.

For example, it is not unusual to find that large areas of skin slough off in the demented. The major reason for this is that it is so difficult to maintain proper hydration in the elderly infirm. Dementia patients, in particular, do not sense and report thirst as would normally be expected, and it's difficult to make someone drink when they feel no need to do so. Because of this, the dementia patient's skin dries and suffers. But coconut oil applied to the skin's surface helps cells seal in the vital moisture needed to maintain skin integrity, as discussed in Chapter 12.

Coconut oil also keeps the areas surrounding toenails and fingernails healthy while inhibiting the growth of opportunistic bacteria and fungi that result in nail thickening and the difficulty of keeping them trimmed and clean.

Coconut oil is soothing to chapped and cracked lips that develop when loved ones lose their normal impulse to hold the mouth in a closed position.

It is helpful in cleanups, too, when normal soap and water might prove too abrasive to get the job done. Lest you think this idea is a bit far fetched, there is nothing that tears more easily or horrifyingly than the fragile skin of a demented elder. Even the skin of a newborn baby is infinitely more resilient. As an antiseptic cleanser, coconut oil is a gentle and welcome friend.

In Lewy body dementia, one of the notable early symptoms is, incredibly, an inconceivably runny nose. My mother would easily go through an entire carton of facial tissues in a day, which sadly is exceedingly rough on a nose. A light application of coconut oil can ease the discomfort of a raw nose and calm inflamed nasal passages, too!

With incontinence and constipation come other special problems. Rashes, vaginal yeast infections, and jock itch are notable among the issues that crop up when elders may become damp or soiled overnight, and coconut oil aids in prevention by providing a nourishing barrier on the skin that inhibits fungal and bacterial growth. In the case of constipation, coconut oil in the diet is a good preventative. But after the fact, when an enema may become necessary, coconut oil is an excellent mild lubricant for easy, pain-free insertion of the syringe.

Finally, when patients become bedridden, everything becomes far more complicated. Coconut oil is excellent for use in light massage to improve circulation, for muscle and nerve stimulation, and as an aid in the prevention of contractures. Furthermore, if your loved one lives long enough in a bed-bound condition, it is likely that you will witness at least one serious skin breakdown known as a bedsore, or decubitus. Do not despair. I have witnessed coconut oil, in combination with frequent turning, allow for these compromised areas to resume their normal appearance much more rapidly than with any amount of normal turning and nursing care alone.

A Coconut Body Balm to Make

Aromatherapy may seem like alchemy to the uninitiated, but therapeutic blends of essential oils really can help elders in the end stages of dementia. Therapeutic essential oils enhance psychological and physical well-being. By utilizing the art and science of blending them to their greatest synergistic effect, elders can be afforded a substantial amount of relief.

TROPICAL TIP

Regardless of the heroic efforts put forth by medical science, unfortunately there still is no cure for the major neurodegenerative diseases. The sad reality is that in the end stages of dementia, it is common for the patient to be bed-bound, anorexic, oxygen dependent, hypertensive, and incontinent. These patients are also predisposed to depression, anxiety, urinary tract infection, bowel impaction, upper respiratory infection, topical yeast infection, contracture, and pressure wounds (decubitus).

Because the most basic need in life is air, the application of essential oils through the olfactory and respiratory systems is often the easiest, most pleasant, and effective way of applying them. But in the case of an end-stage dementia patient's need for mild muscle and circulatory stimulation and the maintenance and improvement of the skin's integrity, a body balm is often a better answer. Aromatherapeutic body balms are formulated for topical application and gentle local massage, while taking into consideration both the actions of the oils and their aesthetic aromatic properties and compatibilities.

A body balm for an elder's fragile, sensitive skin requires a mild, healing emollient as a carrier base. Because of its unique healing properties and ability to be easily absorbed, virgin coconut oil is the carrier oil of choice. It can be used in gentle massage and can be applied directly to inflamed or compromised areas of the skin. But coconut oil is very thin at skin temperature, and the addition of shea butter will give it a little body to provide a more protective moisture barrier than coconut oil would provide on its own.

In the following formula, the essential oils of lavendin and patchouli will be added to the base to provide additional therapeutic actions. The scents of these oils work well together, with lavendin providing both high and middle-note aromatic qualities and patchouli providing the base notes and acting as an enhancer.

The therapeutic actions of lavendin as the primary essential oil work to alleviate and prevent abscesses, blisters, cystitis (urinary bladder infection), dry skin, muscle aches, fatigue, and skin wounds. Patchouli's ability to soothe mature skin and ease stress makes it a good choice to complement the primary essential oil's actions and the carrier oils' attributes.

You will need the following ingredients:

>   1 oz. shea butter
>
>   4 oz. virgin coconut oil
>
>   2 oz. distilled water
>
>   6 ml lavendin essential oil
>
>   .75 ml (37 drops) patchouli essential oil

Here are the steps:

1. Very gently, melt shea butter in a double boiler on a stovetop over medium-low heat.

2. When shea butter has completely melted, remove from heat.

3.   Add coconut oil and distilled water to shea butter and stir.

4.   As mixture begins to cool and thicken, stir in premeasured lavendin essential oil and patchouli essential oil.

5.   Store finished balm covered in an airtight, dark-colored glass container at room temperature.

This body balm preparation will be warming and calming. A very small amount thins out surprisingly to cover a generous area. It is soothing to irritated and dry skin, and on areas prone to decubitus it helps to prevent breakdown of the skin. Any areas prone to yeast will usually resolve within a couple of days.

The Least You Need to Know

- Coconut oil nourishes the brain and nervous tissues of those who suffer from neurodegenerative diseases with ketones when insulin resistance makes them unable to use glucose as fuel.
- Statin and anticholinergic drugs are dangerous to brain and nervous system health and severely exacerbate the symptoms of dementia.
- Many elders have problems with malnutrition due to malabsorption. Coconut oil in the diet helps elders to more efficiently assimilate other nutrients from their diet while also reducing painful sugar cravings.
- Coconut oil has many useful topical applications—especially for the end-stage dementia patient and the bedridden elderly.

Thyroid Function

In This Chapter

- Escalating thyroid disease
- Introducing soy: the incredible, inedible bean
- Undoing the damage

Thyroid disease—primarily hypo- and hyperthyroidism—is among the most prevalent yet underdiagnosed glandular conditions today. In modern times, incidences of thyroid disorders are increasing dramatically and becoming quite widespread.

This chapter attempts to answer the question of why thyroid disease has made such a remarkable rebound in the population and proposes why coconut oil may be part of the new solution.

What Is Thyroid Disease?

The thyroid gland is one of several glands in the endocrine system. It gets its name from the Greek word *thyreoiedes*—shield shaped. More familiarly, however, it is described as being a butterfly-shaped gland located at the base of the neck in front of the trachea and below the Adam's apple.

The glands of the endocrine system control many of the body's functions through the secretion of hormones. These hormones circulate in the bloodstream and work to regulate functions of specific systems in the body. The thyroid gland is integral in controlling how rapidly the body uses energy. It also plays a role in protein production and controls the body's sensitivity to other hormones. Diseases of the thyroid gland directly affect the body's energy, metabolism, growth, weight, and temperature. Thyroid disease has become a very common endocrine disorder, especially in women. There are many forms of thyroid disease, but two are of particular interest.

Hypothyroidism, or underactive thyroid, is a disorder in which the thyroid produces less hormone than is necessary for normal bodily functions. Symptoms include, but are not limited to, the following:

- Thinning hair
- Brittle nails
- Weight gain
- Puffiness in the face
- Chronic fatigue
- A decreased heart rate
- Constipation
- Sensitivity to cold
- Dry skin

Hyperthyroidism, also known as *thyroid toxicosis*, is a disorder in which the thyroid produces more thyroid hormone than is necessary. Symptoms include, but are not limited to, the following:

- Weight loss
- Rapid heart rate
- Bulging eyes
- Nervousness or agitation
- Frequent bowel movements
- Excessive perspiration
- Menstrual irregularities

To help determine whether you may be suffering from a thyroid disorder, you can take the Thyroid Health Quiz in Chapter 1. If you have concerns, your doctor will use several techniques to confirm or rule out a diagnosis. He will take a history, and after assessing your complaints, he will examine your skin, hair, and nails. He will palpate your neck to feel for whether the thyroid gland is enlarged or abnormal feeling. He also will order blood work to determine whether you have appropriate levels of the hormones TSH, T3, and T4 (discussed in the next section) circulating in your blood.

Causes of Thyroid Disease

The production of thyroid hormones is regulated by another hormone: thyroid-stimulating hormone (TSH). TSH is produced by the pituitary gland, which resides deep within the brain. Although it is relatively rare, problems involving the pituitary gland can sometimes be at the root of thyroid disease. Another possible cause for thyroid-related problems is when the liver is unable to transform the T4 hormone into its active form, T3.

A final common cause of thyroid disease is related to insufficient amounts of iodine in the diet, which results in hypothyroidism and sometimes *goiter.*

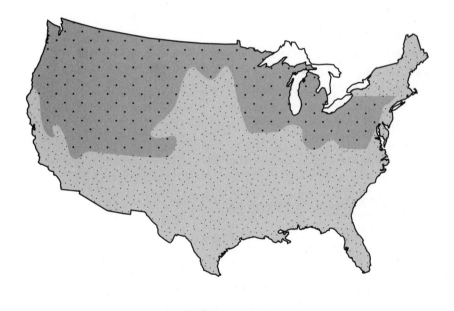

American Goiter Belt

The American goiter belt is a region consisting of iodine-deficient soils.

In the area surrounding the Great Lakes region of the United States, an enlarged thyroid condition known as goiter was quite a problem during the early twentieth century. It became particularly evident during World War I, when many people from Wisconsin and Northern Michigan were disqualified from military service due to the disorder.

The subsequent introduction of sodium iodine to table salt (iodized salt), however, seemed to solve much of the problem. Incidences of goiter and other thyroid problems became relatively rare—until now.

> **DEFINITION**
>
> **Goiter** is the unnatural enlargement of the thyroid gland. This can occur when the thyroid is producing either too much hormone or too little, sometimes even when it is producing the correct amount (called euthyroidism). Goiter indicates that some condition exists that is causing the thyroid gland to grow abnormally.

Low dietary iodine levels alone, however, cannot explain the current increase in hypothyroidism. Iodized salt has been around for decades, and a person really has to search to find table salt that does not have sodium iodine added to it. Furthermore, for quite some time, nutritionists have been encouraging people to increase their consumption of seafood—and seafoods, too, contain appreciable amounts of iodine. In some sectors macrobiotic diets are in vogue, and Asian cuisine is enjoying great popularity as well—both of these dietary traditions offer foods that contain a variety of kelp and seaweed that are full of iodine and other healthy minerals.

Oxidative Stress

By now, nearly everyone is familiar with the notion of free radicals, and many researchers are leaning in that direction when they discuss possible causes of the increase in hypothyroidism. In particular, chemicals and toxins that exist in our water supply and in the soil that our food grows in have become suspect.

Over the years, we have polluted our soil and water with chemical fertilizers, herbicides, fungicides, and pesticides, which are taken up by the plants and animals we eat. By the same token, modern agricultural practices have stripped vital supportive minerals such as selenium from the soil. Certain mining practices release harmful substances into the environment that are known to lower thyroid function as well.

Fluoride and mercury are also tough on the thyroid and inhibit its ability to function. Fluoride is a component of nearly every toothpaste and is found in the drinking water of many communities. Mercury, one of the most toxic metals known to man, is a dynamic component of amalgam fillings in most peoples' mouths. Furthermore, mercury has the ability to displace the selenium eaten in the diet, and selenium is key in converting the thyroid hormone T4 into its active form, T3.

Finally, much of the oxidative stress that the thyroid endures comes from the oils we consume. On his website RayPeat.com, Dr. Ray Peat explains that unsaturated oils (or PUFAs) spontaneously oxidize when they are warm and exposed to oxygen, and when stored in our tissues, they are much warmer and exposed to much more oxygen than they would be in their normal seed state. He goes on to say that the enzymes required for digesting proteins are inhibited by PUFA oils, too.

TO YOUR HEALTH!

Dr. Ray Peat, a physiologist who has studied hormones since 1968, says that the sudden surge of polyunsaturated oils in the food supply since World War II is the culprit for the epidemic of thyroid disease, stating that PUFAs' best understood effect is how much they interfere with the thyroid gland's function.

The inability for these enzymes to function properly disrupts thyroid hormones, which ultimately increases the risk for abnormal blood clotting, inflammation, obesity, and cancer, while simultaneously decreasing available thyroid hormones. Furthermore, since unsaturated oils effectively block protein digestion in the stomach, people can easily become malnourished even while consuming an otherwise healthy diet.

Goitrogens and Soy Oil

Beyond the aforementioned factors, there is one more that has a detrimental effect on thyroid function—the consumption of foods that are classified as *goitrogens*.

DEFINITION

Goitrogens are substances that suppress the thyroid gland's function by hindering iodine uptake. This can cause a goiter, or an enlargement of the thyroid.

Generally speaking, two categories of foods are associated with the disruption of thyroid hormone production—certain legumes like soybeans and their by-products, and cruciferous vegetables. There are a few others, but none of those plays a huge role in our diets.

Dietary Goitrogens

Major Goitrogens	Minor Goitrogens	Insignificant Goitrogens
Peanut products	Broccoli	Millet
Soy products	Brussels sprouts	Peaches
	Cabbage	Radishes
	Cauliflower	Spinach
	Kale	Strawberries
	Kohlrabi	
	Mustard (greens)	
	Turnips	

On the other hand, soy has become ubiquitous in the Western diet. People have been encouraged to increase their consumption of soy and soy products because, we are told, the Japanese, who have lower rates of certain cancers and milder symptoms of menopause, consume lots of soy. This is only a half-truth, though. The Japanese have never consumed soy in the way that we do. The Japanese consume fermented soy products in the form of tofu, soy sauce, miso, and tamari. But until very recently, soybeans and their by-products were always considered inedible. In fact, just a few decades ago, in all of Asia, the soybean was still considered unfit to eat.

Chinese records from the Chou Dynasty (1134–246 B.C.E.) show that the soybean was designated as one of "the five sacred grains." Yet the ancient pictograph that depicted soybean indicates that it was not used as a food. The literature from that period explains that soybeans were used in crop rotation as a means of fixing nitrogen in the soil.

It was in the later part of the second century B.C.E. that methods of fermenting soybeans were discovered. Some of the first fermented soy products included natto, miso, and soy sauce. Eventually, it was discovered that cooked, puréed soybeans could be processed further using magnesium sulfate or calcium sulfate to create soy curd, or tofu. Eventually this method of preparing tofu spread to the rest of Asia, including Japan. Traditionally, though, the Japanese only eat a small amount of tofu or miso in a meal—usually as part of a mineral-rich fish broth, which is followed by a dish that contains some meat or fish.

Unfermented soybeans contain large quantities of natural toxins. These toxins inhibit the enzymes that are needed for protein digestion. The toxins in soybeans are not deactivated by cooking. In addition to reducing our ability to digest proteins, these same toxins are also capable of producing painful gastric disturbances and reducing the uptake of amino acids, too.

DEFINITION

Amino acids are the building blocks of proteins that are essential to tissue building and repair. There are 20 naturally occurring amino acids in foods. Eight of those are essential in the diet and cannot be synthesized by the body.

So soy, besides being goitrogenic and acting directly to reduce thyroid function, introduces many stressors into our diets. Soybeans also contain *haemagglutinin*, a clot-promoting substance that causes red blood cells to clump together, which increases the risk of heart attack or ischemic stroke. And soybeans are extremely high in *phytic acid* content, which blocks the uptake of essential minerals like zinc, calcium, magnesium, copper, and iron.

Increasing Metabolism and Accelerating Thermogenesis

By simply avoiding the most potent goitrogens, you can greatly improve thyroid function and thereby increase your metabolism. Increased metabolism is associated with a sense of increased energy, improved mood and memory, and weight reduction—all the things that people who suffer from poor thyroid function hope for and dream about.

The goitrogens found in soy products are everywhere, though, and they are not always easy to recognize. Soybeans and soy emulsifiers, flours, textured proteins, and shortenings are transformed beyond recognition into infant formulas, plastic-like cheese that won't melt, and the oil your canned tuna swims in. Food manufacturers can even produce sausage-like objects that appear to be hotdogs from soybeans and pretty yellow curds that resemble freshly scrambled eggs.

The following table lists some of the most common names for soy products and the by-products you are likely to find listed on the nutrition information labels of processed foods.

Foods to Avoid for Improved Thyroid Health

Soy Products	Soy Ingredients	Soy-Containing Food
Soybean oil	Soy protein	Vegetable broths
Edamame	Soy protein isolate	Worcestershire sauce
Soy milk	Hydrolized protein	Baked goods
Soy sprouts	Natural flavoring	Infant formulas
Tofu	Artificial flavor	Miso
Textured vegetable protein (TVP)		Soy sauce
Soy flour		Tamari
		Tempeh
		Canned fish

By far, however, we encounter the most soy in the form of soybean oil—often only identified as "vegetable oil." Look at the ingredients label of any processed, fried, or baked foods and you almost certainly will find soybean oil listed. To make matters worse, it will probably be "partially hydrogenated" as well.

By avoiding processed foods and by replacing vegetable oils with coconut oil in your diet, you can reduce the oxidative stress imposed by PUFAs and avoid exposure to goitrogens at the same time! Because coconut oil is saturated and very stable, it does not cause the oxidative stress on tissues like unsaturated vegetable oils do. Because coconut oil does not inhibit the enzymes that are integral for T4-to-T3 conversion in the liver, the thyroid gland does not have to work as hard. Because coconut oil is instantly converted to fuel, it also enhances thermogenesis, which in turn enhances energy and contributes to weight loss.

The following are several simple changes you can make in your habits to improve thyroid function and metabolism:

- Replace all cooking oils with coconut oil.
- Learn to identify soy products and read every label on packaged foods.
- Make your own salad dressings and mayonnaise using coconut oil (see Chapter 16).
- Avoid restaurant meals, which usually are full of trans-fats and vegetable oils that have been heated to very high temperatures.
- Experiment with smoothies and other recipes that deliciously incorporate coconut oil (see Chapters 15 to 17).
- Eat iodine-rich foods, especially seafood, sea salt, and kelp.
- Exercise. Exercise stimulates the thyroid gland and increases the body's sensitivity to thyroid hormones.
- Along the same lines, learn and practice an inverted yoga posture such as *Sarvangasana*, the candle pose. Poses like these create increased blood flow to the thyroid gland, enhancing thyroid health and function.

The Least You Need to Know

- In recent years, the incidence of thyroid disease has increased beyond anything that can be accounted for by iodine deficiency alone.
- The thyroid gland is sensitive to dietary and environmental stressors and toxins.
- Soybeans, soybean oil, and soy by-products are powerful goitrogens. They are everywhere in the modern Western diet and do substantial damage to the thyroid's ability to function and our ability to assimilate nutrients from our diets.
- Removing unfermented soy products from our diets and replacing soybean oil with coconut oil will relieve stress on the thyroid gland, increase the uptake of available nutrition, increase metabolism, and promote the loss of excess weight.

Weight Loss and Maintenance

In This Chapter

- Discovering why low-carb dieting is healthy
- Learning the big fat advantage—literally
- Preventing the wasting of lean body tissues
- Heart-healthy saturated fat

Low-carbohydrate weight-loss diets have enjoyed quite a resurgence of popularity in recent decades. Heralded by the republication of the 1992 bestseller *Dr. Atkins' New Diet Revolution*, countless other diet books such as Dr. Barry Sears's *The Zone Diet*, Dr. Arthur Agatston's *The South Beach Diet*, and Dr. Pierre Dukan's *The Dukan Diet* have followed in rapid succession. The reason all these diets have enjoyed so much success? They work. Moreover, they work while improving overall health. This chapter is going to explain how fats can be your ally in weight loss and management.

Low-Carb Dieting with Coconut Oil

Recent 2001 research shows that diets containing medium-chain triglycerides (MCTs), like those found in coconut oil, result in the storage of less body fat than diets without them. One such study looked at the consumption of MCTs as compared to that of other fats in healthy adults with healthy body weights. In this study, the carbohydrate and protein consumption of the subjects were equal. Results demonstrated that MCT fats helped to increase weight loss by reducing body fat significantly more than other fats did. In 2003, a similar study was published that looked at moderately overweight men consuming diets rich in MCTs. This study showed an even greater reduction in body fat than the 2001 study, along with an increase in the subjects' ability to burn calories from normal activity.

As discussed in Chapter 10, one key to MCTs' effect on weight loss seems to be thermogenesis. Diet-induced thermogenesis is an increase in calorie expenditure due to the body's production of heat that occurs after meals—otherwise known as the *thermic effect* of food. This is a huge advantage to folks who are trying to lose weight.

While diet-induced thermogenesis is not as powerful a weight-loss determinant as the *basal metabolic rate* or *activity-induced thermogenesis*, it plays an important role in the body's makeup. The increased thermic effect of consuming the MCTs in coconut oil means excess calories are less likely to end up stored as body fat. They are rapidly converted to energy instead.

DEFINITION

Basal metabolic rate is the rate at which calories are used up in the regulation of normal bodily functions—while sleeping, for example.

Activity-induced thermogenesis is heat energy fueled by the calories consumed in any activity, such as housekeeping, walking, or riding a bicycle.

Because MCTs help increase metabolism, coconut oil is a perfect adjunct to a healthy, low-carbohydrate, weight-loss diet.

Furthermore, while low-carbohydrate diets are famous for producing a sense of satiation, the consumption of medium-chain, fatty-acid-rich coconut oil enhances that effect. Greater satiety means less hunger and fewer cravings, which makes staying on any weight-reduction program more doable.

Eat Fat to Lose Fat?

According to NHANES, the National Health and Nutrition Examination Survey (Flegal, et al. 2012), in the United States:

- 68.8 percent of adults are overweight; of those, 35.7 percent are *obese* and 5.4 percent are *morbidly obese.*

- 31.8 percent of children and adolescents are overweight, and 16.9 percent of those are obese.

DEFINITION

Obese people are those whose *body mass index* (BMI) is 30 or greater. Obesity results from an abnormal accumulation of body fat and is associated with increased risk of illness, disability, and death.

Morbidly obese people weigh two or more times their ideal weight and have a BMI of 40 to 49.9. This condition is associated with many serious and life-threatening disorders.

Body mass index (BMI) is determined by using one of the following formulas.

- English: BMI = [weight in pounds $\div$ (height in inches)^2]$\times$ 703
- Metric: BMI = weight in kilograms $\div$ (height in meters)^2

If you are among the growing number of overweight or obese, and you have tried dieting and exercise with little or no success, you may be on the wrong diet—the frequently prescribed, low-calorie, high-carbohydrate, "less than 30 percent fat" diet. The low-fat diet is, in large part, what's at the root of our current obesity epidemic. Yet the advice that says, "in order to lose weight you must follow a low-fat diet," has been drilled so deeply into the modern psyche that most people would believe it is a scientifically proven fact. Unfortunately for those who are futilely struggling to lose weight using this dictum, the science proves something quite the opposite.

Obesity is caused by a particular type of *malnutrition* that triggers a specific metabolic defect. That's right—obesity is a symptom of malnutrition, is not a disease, and is not necessarily the result of poor willpower or a lack of discipline.

You may recall from earlier discussions about Dr. Ian Prior's and Dr. Weston A. Price's research that neither ever found a group of primitive people following an indigenous diet that was purely vegetarian. To the contrary, they found many peoples who ate little or no plant material and appeared to be "health and vitality" personified.

Now, I am not going to tell you that there is something wrong with eating fruits and vegetables because that is certainly not the case. Vegetables and fruits, especially in their natural states, are some of the most nutritious and beneficial foods on earth. But what I will tell you is that omitting natural fat from your diet—while allowing sweets, highly processed grain products (flours, polished rice, noodles, etc.), and polyunsaturated or hydrogenated vegetable oils— will lead directly to problems of being overweight. And because of how insulin behaves in the body, this sort of low-fat diet is doomed to fail—even if you are restricting calories!

The Fat Advantage

Fortunately, not everyone has taken the low-fat, low-calorie propaganda hook, line, and sinker. Researchers in Germany, among others, have done the world quite a service by looking into the metabolic advantage afforded by fats over carbohydrates. An example of such research is a study conducted at the University of Würzburg and published in 1978.

In this study, 45 dieters were studied for 5 weeks. Each patient was placed on a strict 1,000-calorie diet. Approximately half of the dieters were placed on a low-fat version, while the other half were on a low-carbohydrate version of the diet. The results showed a significant metabolic advantage to the low-carbohydrate diet in that the low-carb dieters averaged 9.24 pounds of weight loss over and above that which was lost by the low-fat dieters. Robert Atkins, MD, describes how this is possible in his book *Dr. Atkins' New Diet Revolution* when he discusses a patient he calls Harry.

Dr. Atkins' patient, Harry, had been gaining a pound every two weeks, which meant Harry was eating 250 calories per day over the amount he needed—totaling a daily average caloric intake of 2,129 calories.

When Harry switched to the low-carbohydrate diet, he lost 3.9 pounds per week on average. According to the caloric restriction theory of weight loss, Harry would have had to reduce his caloric intake by 1,950 calories per day to achieve this. Given the fact that he was gaining a half-pound per week on 2,129 calories, his breakeven point would have been 1,879 calories per day.

So in order to lose 3.9 pounds per week, he would have had to take in 1,950 less than 1,879 calories—or a grand total of –71 calories! That's right: $1,879 - 1,950 = -71$.

If the caloric theory of weight loss worked, Harry would have to have been eating less than nothing—a clear impossibility. In actuality, Harry was consuming 49 calories each day more than his "break-even" point of 1,879 and should have gained 1.3 pounds over the 13 weeks of his low-carb diet instead of losing 50.

By eschewing refined carbohydrates and making dietary proteins and fats the basis of his diet, Harry discovered what Dr. Atkins refers to as a "metabolic advantage"—and a substantial one at that. Anything Harry ate above the –71 calories while he continued to lose weight is an incredible metabolic advantage indeed, and in Harry's case that amounted to 1,999 calories per day.

High-carbohydrate diets, especially those that contain foods high on the *glycemic index*, require large amounts of the insulin hormone that is necessary for getting glucose into your cells. With continual spiking and crashing of sugar and the resultant insulin in your bloodstream comes insulin resistance. When sugar is unable to get into and fuel your cells, your body stores the excess energy as fat. All this comes together to form a vicious downward spiral, leading to continued weight gain, greater insulin resistance, metabolic syndrome including hypoglycemia, and eventually diabetes. And it's all because of consuming a malnourishing diet that is imbalanced with respect to fat and carbohydrate intake.

DEFINITION

The **glycemic index** is a measure of the rate and level of glucose (blood sugar) increase resulting from food consumption.

While a body uses glucose to fuel its cells, it doesn't necessarily need to get its fuel from food. If you stop consuming high-carbohydrate foods that trigger the insulin response, your body will begin *lipolysis*—melting your excess fat away to produce ketones that provide the necessary fuel. This is a process known as benign dietary ketosis, or keto-lipolysis.

This is a survival mechanism as old as the human race itself. Without the ability to convert stored body fat into ketones for use as energy, primitive man would never have survived his first drought or famine. Therefore, low-carbohydrate, ketogenic diets are truly nature's answer to achieving and maintaining perfect body weight. And including healthy MCTs in your diet, in the form of coconut oil, only serves to augment the effect.

What If I Need to Gain Weight?

If you think achieving weight loss is a problem, imagine the possibility of not being able to gain weight or, in fact, continually losing weight regardless of the amount of food you consume. Some unfortunate people don't have to imagine this because they deal with the stark reality every day.

Fortunately, MCTs have been found to be helpful with cachexia—a *wasting* syndrome associated with uncontrollable weight loss. Cachexia is most often thought of as being "wasting secondary to cancer." In his fascinating book *Beating Cancer with Nutrition*, Patrick

Quillin points out that more cancer patients actually die due to starvation than cancer. But cachexia is also seen in conditions such as cystic fibrosis, Crohn's disease, the dementias, certain pancreatic disorders, AIDS, and many others.

> **DEFINITION**
>
> **Wasting** refers to the fact that the body will consume itself under dire conditions of malnutrition. It will eat up its own muscle tissue and so on in order to survive when nutrients are unavailable, stolen by cancers or parasites, or under other extremely taxing conditions. Wasting's tragic end is ultimately starvation after the body has consumed all of its stored reserves of nutrition.

Among the many reasons for uncontrolled weight loss are conditions that result in the malabsorption of nutrients. These conditions are seen in the elderly, in end-stage dementia patients, and in diseases of the gallbladder and pancreas where there are insufficient enzymes or other factors available to absorb and assimilate the nutrients in food. Because of their unique medium-chain structure, the fatty acids found in coconut oil can benefit anyone who is unable to properly utilize long-chain fats. The MCTs found in coconut oil have even proven particularly useful for nourishing premature babies whose digestive systems are still underdeveloped.

A study published in 1991 in the *Journal of Nutrition* describes how baby pigs were able to absorb these shorter-chain fatty acids with significantly greater ease than the longer-chain polyunsaturates, which confirms their use in infant formulas. But elders, indeed anyone with a decreased ability to absorb dietary nutrition, can benefit greatly as well.

Cancer Care

As Dr. Quillin attested, because starvation is the tragic end of so many cancer patients, it becomes obvious that dietary choices in the care of cancer patients are particularly crucial. Some studies show that a low-carbohydrate, ketogenic diet with the addition of MCTs like coconut oil can help inhibit the growth of tumors.

You may be thinking, "Wait a minute! Didn't she just say that ketogenic diets result in weight loss?" Well, that is true, but only if there is *excess fat* to lose. Ketogenic diets do not cause wasting of vital tissues. On a ketogenic diet, muscle is preserved and can, in fact, be built, while only excess fat is converted into ketones for energy.

Treating Cachexia (Wasting Secondary to Cancer)

Interesting research has been conducted using MCT-based ketogenic diets for the treatment of cancer in particular. Some of these studies have shown that a low-carbohydrate, ketogenic diet that includes the MCTs of coconut oil significantly inhibits tumor growth in mice. In 1995, a study was published in the *Journal of the American Dietetic Association* that followed pediatric patients with advanced cancers. This study showed that MCT-based ketogenic diets slowed tumor growth while increasing metabolism.

In addition to their ability to inhibit tumor growth, however, MCTs also show the potential to fight the cachexia that cancers cause. Cancer cells love sugar—and they are greedy! They are capable of consuming up to 15 times more glucose than noncancerous cells. In cachexia secondary to cancer, the cancer cells go merrily along gorging on all the glucose they can get their hands on, while healthy tissue starves and devastating weight loss results. One British study following veterinary colon cancer patients who had been placed on a high-MCT ketogenic diet found that not only were tumor sizes reduced, but that weight loss was reduced as well!

Because a ketogenic diet drastically reduces the sugar available to cancer cells, inhibiting their growth while providing ketones to fuel normal cells and bodily functions, these exciting studies suggest that high-MCT, low-carbohydrate, ketogenic diets may be the best tool for staving off the dangers of wasting syndromes that are so often the determining factor in whether a cancer is fatal.

Advantages for Athletes

The MCTs of coconut oil are also an invaluable asset to weight lifters and other athletes who severely restrict carbohydrates during intensive training. Coconut oil's MCTs provide ketones that bypass the need for glucose metabolism while they fuel the muscles and aid in the process of muscle recovery.

Adequate protein consumption is vitally important to athletes as well. Since MCTs are quickly converted into energy, they prevent the body from using amino acids and proteins as fuel. This allows vital dietary proteins to be used to their greatest advantage—in the building and repair of muscle tissue.

Furthermore, without this ketone advantage and with little body fat to spare, the athlete's body would begin to break down its own muscle tissues during intensive training to satisfy its energy needs. The ketones provided by the MCTs in coconut oil spare athletes from catabolic muscle wasting while fueling cells and making protein available for muscle building and repair.

Do Saturated Fats Clog Arteries and Raise Cholesterol?

The major arguments against low-carbohydrate diets have always involved the notion that a diet high in protein and fat would be dangerous to cardiovascular health. It is interesting to note, however, that the major proponents of the low-carb diet are cardiologists. It turns out that Dr. Atkins and Dr. Agatston turned to the low-carb approach to dieting in order to improve their patients' heart health—and with stellar results.

Low-carbohydrate diets, properly followed, do not clog arteries or raise cholesterol. They do, however, result in the following heart-healthy outcomes:

- High blood pressure will come down.
- Insulin levels will stabilize.

- High blood sugar will be reduced and stabilize.
- Triglyceride levels will rapidly and profoundly plummet.
- Serum cholesterol levels will come down.

This, of course, is not to mention the fact that you will lose excess weight, which in and of itself is a significant contribution to the health of your heart—and your health in general.

Chapter 13 further discusses how coconut oil benefits the heart and arteries. For a full treatment of all the advantages of a low-carbohydrate diet and why it is a healthy diet for the cardiovascular system, I recommend Dr. Atkins's books (see Appendix B). Together, low-carb dieting augmented with the MCTs of coconut oil form a formidable tool for the improvement and preservation of cardiovascular health.

The Least You Need to Know

- Low-carb dieting is an effective, heart-healthy method of weight loss and maintenance, and coconut oil augments results.
- Coconut oil is useful in cases of wasting diseases as well. Cancer patients, premature infants, and athletes can all use coconut oil to their advantage.
- Naturally saturated fats like those found in coconut oil do not raise cholesterol or clog arteries.

Healthy Skin and Hair

In This Chapter

- Applying coconut oil, both inside and out
- Tapping into tropical skincare
- Using synergistic sunlight, coconut oil, and vitamin D
- Understanding the properties that fight inflammation and odor

For many thousands of years, coconut oil has been used to keep skin soft and smooth. In the tropics it is also highly valued for its ability to give hair a healthful, lustrous shine. Women from Polynesia and India are world renown for their lovely skin and hair despite year-round exposure to a sun declination that would challenge the hardiest of human beings. Research shows that the traditional use of coconut oil in these parts of the world is responsible for these stellar results.

Coconut oil works to nourish the skin and hair from two different avenues. It works internally by supporting the nutrition that is necessary for the building of healthy skin and hair tissue, and it works externally when applied to skin and hair to protect and maintain its healthy condition. Natural coconut oil has a small molecular structure that is easily absorbed by the skin. While it is soothing and moisturizing on its own, it is also an excellent addition to other body-care products like soaps, ointments, lip balms, lotions, and conditioners.

Protection from the Sun

Many of the skin-care products people use are actually damaging to the skin. They contain a variety of chemicals, dyes, alcohol, and synthetic fragrances that not only damage the surface of the skin, but are absorbed and do more damage inside the body.

According to Dr. Bruce Fife of the Coconut Research Center, coconut oil has been used as a natural sunscreen and skin protectant in tropical climates for thousands of years.

He explains that, in Polynesia, the oil was regarded as sacred, and although the islanders wore little clothing in order to keep cool, they did not suffer skin-damaging sunburns because of their liberal use of coconut oil. Women of Polynesia would slather their babies with coconut oil soon after giving birth. Every day mothers would continue to apply coconut oil to their children until they were able to do so themselves, and they would maintain this daily ritual until the day they died.

Privy to this information, manufacturers of the first commercial suntan lotions used coconut oil as one of their main ingredients. Coconut oil has an amazing ability to protect the skin without blocking UV radiation from the sun. This is important because fats are necessary for the absorption of fat-soluble vitamins (A, D, E, and K) and in the creation of vitamin D in the skin. Vitamins A, D, and E, in particular, are marvelously potent antioxidants and are key to the health of skin and hair.

Preventing Wrinkles and Dry Skin

Technically speaking, vitamin D does not fit the classic definition of a vitamin. It is not a substance we can readily get in sufficient quantities from food sources. Functionally speaking, vitamin D is a hormone that is synthesized in the skin. The skin has the ability to manufacture as much as 10,000 IU of vitamin D after only 20 to 30 minutes of sun exposure at an optimal declination of the sun.

You can begin to see how, in the tropics with direct light from the sun, all the key ingredients for youthful skin come together in a beautiful synergy. The fat of coconut oil is present both on the skin's surface and internally because of habitual consumption. This fat is key to the absorption of vitamin D, which can only be manufactured in the skin with sufficient sun exposure.

TO YOUR HEALTH!

The angle of the sun is important because, at 42°N Latitude (or higher), the angle of the sun is too oblique in wintertime for the synthesis of vitamin D. During winter, the sun stays low on the horizon and its rays do not reach Earth in a very direct manner, giving us more of a glancing "blow."

Areas in the continental United State at 42°N Latitude include Detroit, Michigan; Chicago, Illinois; the California/Oregon border; the Idaho/Nevada border; the New York/Pennsylvania border; Cape Cod, Massachusetts; and Rhode Island.

Vitamin D's Role

Calcitriol, the active form of vitamin D, is one of the most powerful hormones known. It has the ability to activate more than 2,000 genes. But before vitamin D can become calcitriol, it first undergoes a complex series of changes that begin in the outermost layer of the skin, the epidermis, and this is key to the skin having a youthful appearance.

Cholesterol, which plays many important roles in the body, is integral to the formation of vitamin D. In the skin, a type of cholesterol (7-dehydrocholesterol) is activated by ultraviolet B (UVB) rays from the sun and is converted to vitamin D_3. The vitamin D then travels through the bloodstream to the liver and kidneys, where it is converted to the active vitamin D hormone, 1,25-dihydroxycholecalciferol.

Because vitamin D is fat soluble, it crosses the lipid (fatty) membranes of cells and migrates to the cell's nucleus. There it binds with vitamin D receptors, where it can regulate the expression of genes that turn certain cell functions on or off. Every human cell has vitamin D receptors. Vitamin D receptors in the skin regulate healthy cell proliferation and differentiation, as well as immune function.

Coconut oil, the sun, and vitamin D work together to maintain the skin's integrity. This is a vitally important job since the skin is the body's first line of defense against germs, yeast, and other invaders, and it must also be replaced at a rate of nearly 40,000 cells per minute!

Wouldn't Any Oil Do?

Here is where you might think that any oil or fat may accomplish the same function as coconut oil in the manufacture of vitamin D in the skin. But that is not the case. All fats are not equal. Unsaturated fats tend to become rancid and introduce free radicals to the skin. Unsaturated fats such as canola or soybean oil also reduce the binding of vitamin D, while the 92-percent saturated fat of coconut oil enhances this crucial binding activity that enables the skin cells to divide and differentiate. This cell activity in the *keratinocytes* of the epidermis is responsible for maintaining the delicate structure, or matrix, of the skin tissue. It forms an integral barrier that locks in moisture to keep the skin soft and smooth. Without this activity, the skin becomes thin and fragile. Dryness and wrinkling set in as moisture is lost and cells are unable to be replaced.

DEFINITION

A **keratinocyte** is any one of the cells in the skin that synthesize keratin. **Keratin** is a durable protein polymer found only in epithelial cells. It provides the structural strength to the skin, hair, and nails.

Youthful, Shiny Hair

Keratin is integral to the structure and strength of hair as well as that of the skin, so what coconut oil does for the skin, it can do for the hair, too.

Washing our skin or hair with detergents, soaps, and shampoos removes the natural protective barrier of *sebum*. This leaves hair vulnerable to sun, wind, and chemical damage. It also reduces the strength and resilience of hair.

To remain beautiful and strong, hair has an even greater need for protection from the elements than the skin because hair is not alive. While healthy skin has the ability to replace damaged or dying cells with new tissue, once a shaft of hair is damaged, its structure cannot be repaired in the same way. A healthy head of hair depends on healthy scalp tissue and the protective barrier afforded by sebum.

> **DEFINITION**
>
> **Sebum** is the oily secretion (made up of keratin, fat, and cellular debris) of the sebaceous glands of the skin. It forms a moist, acidic film that is mildly antifungal and antibacterial and protects the skin and hair against drying.

Coconut oil applied to the scalp promotes the healthy scalp tissue that hair depends on. Applied directly to the hair itself, it serves as a protective barrier until the body is able to replace the sebum lost in the course of washing. This is important for people who are in the habit of washing their hair daily and for people who suffer from hypothyroidism. In either case, the hair never has a chance to completely regain its normal sebum before the hair is washed and stripped of it again.

In addition to maintaining normal healthy hair, coconut oil can be helpful in treating unpleasant conditions of the scalp and hair as well. Coconut oil can eradicate dandruff and remove cradle cap. Because of its ability to fight fungal infections, it can cure tinea capitis, or ringworm of the scalp. Because it is antibacterial and readily absorbed by the skin, it can prevent folliculitis, an angry infection of the hair follicles that results in the formation of painful boils. Coconut oil has even been used in the prevention and removal of head lice!

Using coconut oil in the hair and on the scalp as a routine hair treatment is easy:

1. After shampooing, take a pea-size or smaller dab of coconut oil and rub it thoroughly into the palms of your hands.

2. Run your hands through the entire length of your hair beginning at the scalp and paying special attention to dry ends.

3. Comb through and style as usual.

The method for deeply conditioning the hair and scalp using coconut oil prior to shampooing is described in Chapter 18.

TROPICAL TIP

Localized infections, such as patches of yeast or fungus, can be ameliorated by topically applying coconut oil directly to the problem spot.

Coconut oil is helpful in the prevention of head lice because its oily nature does not allow the little creatures to easily attach their eggs, or nits, to the hair. If a louse's egg won't stick to the base of the hair shaft, the continuation of its life cycle is effectively terminated. The nits will come out of the hair with normal washing and combing and be lost down the drain or in the waste bin—and if the little egg manages to survive all of that, the louse that emerges will not be in a position to get the blood meal it needs in order to survive.

Getting rid of head lice using coconut oil is a bit more involved than prevention, but it is a far safer process than using toxic pediculicides on your scalp.

TO YOUR HEALTH!

Infections such as head boils, and toxic chemicals placed on the scalp— (peliculicides) like those that kill lice—are particularly worrisome because the tissues that lie above the lip line on the head share return blood flow with the brain. The blood and all the toxins, bacteria, and so on involved in the infection must run back through the brain before being re-oxygenated and put back into circulation in the rest of the body. This endangers the delicate brain tissue which is normally protected from pathogens by what is known as the blood-brain barrier. Although complications are rare, a boil (or other toxins) on or above the lip line, on the nose or scalp, or in the outer ear can be serious because infections and toxins in these areas have easy access to the brain.

Follow these steps to naturally rid the hair of head lice using coconut oil:

1. Completely saturate the hair and scalp with a mixture of 2 tablespoons of coconut oil and 3 to 5 drops of tea tree oil.

2. Cover the treated hair securely with a plastic bag for 12 hours or overnight.

3. Sit in the sunlight until the bag feels warm to the touch. Alternatively, you could heat the hair with a warm hair dryer, being very careful not to melt the bag.

4. Remove the bag and apply 6 ounces of shampoo directly to the hair without wetting it first. Massage into the hair very well.

5. Use the plastic bag to cover the scalp and hair again for about 30 minutes while the oil begins to break down.

6. Rinse your hair as thoroughly as possible. (It will still feel a bit oily.)

7. Comb through the hair to remove tangles.

8. Beginning at the nape of the neck and working over the entire area of the scalp, use a lice-removal comb to remove nits, one small section of hair at a time.

9. Rinse the comb and wipe it with a clean tissue after completing each section.

10. When finished, you can wash the hair again to remove the remaining oil, but know that any lice that may be lurking around will have a harder time attaching nits to oily hair shafts.

Precautions should be taken to ensure bedding and furniture has been thoroughly cleaned and vacuumed (boiled, if possible). Be vigilant to inspect the scalp daily, and repeat the treatment once per week for three more weeks (four treatments in all).

Rashes, Eczema, and Psoriasis

According to research published in the March 1999 issue of *Immunology*, coconut oil possesses a profound anti-inflammatory action. It achieves this by reducing the presence of inflammatory chemicals in the body. This attribute of coconut oil makes it useful in reducing a number of acute and chronic inflammations. On a sensory level, inflammation is indicated by heat, redness, and swelling, all of which are present in rashes.

Some rashes are caused by infections of yeast, fungus, or bacteria. Because coconut oil also has remarkable antifungal and antibacterial properties, topical application of coconut oil not only reduces the uncomfortable inflammation, but also effectively kills the pathogen at the root of the rash. Eczema, contact dermatitis, ringworm, and diaper rash can be relieved or even cleared completely by the application of coconut oil. Psoriasis is an interesting "rash" of another sort, however. Psoriasis is a nonmalignant inflammatory condition in which the proliferation of skins cells far outstrips differentiation.

You will recall from earlier in this chapter that skin cell proliferation and differentiation are in large part controlled by the active form of vitamin D, which is manufactured in the skin upon exposure to sunlight. In fact, for many years, medical doctors have treated inflammatory skin disorders by the application of UV radiation alone. But vitamin D works best and is absorbed more readily in the presence of certain saturated fats.

Dr. Michael D. Holick recognized this and, in his landmark research and double-blind studies of vitamin D, found that psoriasis responds remarkably well to topical application of vitamin D in a base of petroleum jelly. Unfortunately, the strength of the product that he tested and the FDA approved (15 milligrams vitamin D_3/gram-base) is not available in the United States. But you can easily make your own preparation that contains only slightly less vitamin D_3 and has the healthy added benefit of using coconut oil as opposed to being a petroleum-based product.

For this you will need a sensitive electronic kitchen scale that measures in grams and a source of 50,000 IU capsules of vitamin D_3, cholecalciferol. (See the resources in Appendix B for sources of 50,000 IU vitamin D_3 capsules and coconut oil.)

1. Gently heat 100 grams of coconut oil until it melts.

2. Mix in the contents of one 50,000 IU capsule of vitamin D_3. This will result in a 12.5 mcg (microgram) D_3 per gram-base ointment.

3. Pour the mixture into a clean jar and allow it to solidify.

4. Apply topically to affected areas daily.

TO YOUR HEALTH!

You can view an incredibly informative and vastly entertaining medical seminar on this fascinating subject, conducted at the University of California, San Diego by Dr. Michael F. Holick, PhD, MD, online at tiny. cc/6eechw. Dr. Holick is a professor of medicine, physiology, and biophysics at Boston University School of Medicine.

Underarm Deodorizer

To prevent underarm odor, you first have to understand what causes it. Because commercially available deodorants are also typically anti-perspirants, you might be thinking that sweat causes underarm odor. But this is not the case. Sweat is mostly composed of water and salt. It is the action of bacteria that are attracted to warm, moist areas of the skin that produces underarm odor.

Apocrine and eccrine glands are the two kinds of glands that produce sweat. Eccrine glands are found in the palms of the hands and on the plantar surface of the feet. They open directly to the surface of the skin. Apocrine glands, however, are situated in a way that they open into hair follicles. These are the type of glands you have in your underarm area, and they produce a sweat rich with proteins and fatty acids, including a carbohydrate called sialomucin. Sialomucin is a glycoprotein, a protein that has a sugar coating. Because apocrine glands are located in areas that stay warm and moist, these areas can become like an incubator for breeding the kinds of bacteria responsible for body odor.

Yeasts and some types of bacteria really like sweets. So the sugar-coated proteins in your sweat become an ideal food source for them. The bacteria metabolize the sugar either through *anaerobic respiration* or a process of fermentation, and the by-product of the bacteria's energy production is body odor.

DEFINITION

Anaerobic respiration is a form of cellular respiration that occurs when oxygen is scarce or absent.

Different bacteria produce different odors. For example, the bacteria responsible for what is commonly recognized as foot odor are *Staphylococcus epidermidis* and *Bacillus subtilis*. A combination of *Staphylococcus epidermidis* and *Corynebacterium xerosis*, on the other hand, are responsible for odor emitted from sweaty underarms.

The reason commercially available underarm deodorants work is because they make the armpits into a hostile environment for the bacteria that are most likely to live there and multiply. They can't reproduce in appreciable numbers, so body odor remains low. But what if those bacteria weren't there at all? Then there would be no odor either.

The medium-chain fatty acids in coconut oil have special antibacterial properties because they are able to disintegrate bacterial cell walls. In fact, in their search for nontoxic agents to control and disable the new "super bug" strains of bacteria, researchers are discovering that the fatty acids in coconut oil (particularly lauric acid) may be a powerful new tool.

A light application of straight coconut oil to the underarm area—or any other area prone to body odor—will effectively kill off most odor-causing bacteria. It will not stain clothes, and if you're using virgin coconut oil, it will also have a delightfully fresh scent. If, on the other hand, you prefer a more conventional form of deodorant, you can make one yourself using the recipe in Chapter 18.

The Least You Need to Know

- Coconut oil works both inside the body and when topically applied to maintain the healthy and youthful look of skin and hair.

- The routine application of coconut oil by traditional tropical peoples kept their skin and hair youthful, lustrous, and supple into old age.

- Coconut oil and sunlight work synergistically to produce vitamin D in the skin. The skin's own vitamin D receptors work, in turn, to provide the skin with added protection.

- Coconut oil has many anti-inflammatory and antibacterial properties that are useful in calming rashes, killing overgrowths of bacteria, healing psoriasis, and eliminating body odor.

Heart Disease

In This Chapter

- Challenging the saturated fat taboo
- Understanding cholesterol: it's not what you think …
- Making the inflammation connection
- Realizing the politically *in*correct

Throughout this book, the effects of saturated fats on cardiovascular health have been discussed quite a lot, but since saturated fats in the diet have been taboo for so long, their effect on heart health deserves its own chapter. In this chapter you will discover that saturated fats, such as those found in coconut oil, are heart healthy and that many of the things you have been lead to believe about heart health are simply not true.

Dietary Changes Affect Health

As discussed in Chapter 6, the Pukapuka and Tokelau peoples of New Zealand enjoyed excellent health on their native diets, which were high in saturated fat from coconut and, to some extent, from animal fat. But when they migrated to the mainland of New Zealand and adopted a modern diet, their health suffered. So how did their diets change?

The total saturated fats in the islanders' diets actually decreased after the migration—from 50 percent to 41 percent of caloric intake. Strangely, this decrease in saturated fat intake coincided with an increase in LDL (bad) cholesterol and a reduction of HDL (good) cholesterol. Also increasing in the islanders' diets were polyunsaturated fatty acid (PUFA) and sugar. Before moving, 80 percent of islanders' dietary fats came from coconut oil, but afterward, coconut oil only made up 43 percent of the total. Additionally, they consumed more white bread, rice, and other processed Western foods after the move.

According to Dr. Ian A. Prior and others, the Pukapuka and Tokelau islanders enjoyed ideal body weight and serum cholesterol levels as well as freedom from degenerative disease on their traditional high-saturated-fat diets, but their health deteriorated to mirror that of Western cultures as soon as they reduced intake of coconut oil and began consuming PUFAs and other processed modern foods.

Saturated Fat and Cholesterol

You have heard the phrase over and over again: *artery-clogging saturated fat and cholesterol.* But the use of this phrase is completely misleading and obfuscates the truth. The truth is that the fats in the plaques that clog arteries are primarily made up of *un*saturated fats. Yes, you read that right. To be exact, the fats that are components of arterial plaques are composed of 74 percent *un*saturated fat combined with some cholesterol.

You may be asking yourself how this can be. The reason PUFA and monosaturated fats collect in arterial walls is because only oxidized fats and cholesterol end up there. Saturated fats do not easily oxidize because of their stable structure. But unsaturated fats oxidize easily during processing and when exposed to heat.

Furthermore, the cholesterol that ends up in arterial plaques does not necessarily come from saturated fat. It has been determined that consuming saturated fat and cholesterol does not raise blood cholesterol levels, but that the body makes its own cholesterol in response to the body's needs. Cholesterol acts like a patch in the body. It is not the villain running around wreaking havoc. Cholesterol is the paramedic trying to stem the tide of inflammation that causes arterial damage, so that your body does not suffer a blowout in the form of an aneurysm or hemorrhagic stroke.

Finally, the body does not need saturated fat to manufacture cholesterol. Other fats, sugar, and even carbohydrates like those in fruits, vegetables, and grains end up being converted by the liver into cholesterol as your body sees fit. Since cholesterol is integral to the maintenance and repair of body tissues, the body will manufacture it regardless of what you eat. What determines how much and what kind of cholesterol gets made is how much our diets and lifestyles create inflammation and damage tissues in the body.

Blood Clotting Tendencies

Another factor that determines cardiovascular health is the blood's tendency to clot. Clotting, of course, is necessary for survival. If our blood did not clot, even a small bruise or cut would result in our bleeding to death—a frightening proposition. Luckily for us, our blood does clot, and it does so because our blood platelets become sticky.

Normally, when a blood vessel is injured and its endothelial lining is damaged, coagulation begins almost instantly. The injury exposes blood platelets to a protein known as *platelet tissue factor* and initiates a change in the platelets that produces fibrinogen and fibrin proteins in a complex cascade of reactions. The sticky proteins immediately begin forming a mesh to plug up the blood flow at the site of the injury. But when platelets become sticky and adhere to arterial walls, they can form dangerous clots that may block blood flow and result in a heart attack or an ischemic stroke.

When doctors examine the blood qualities of recent heart attack and stroke victims, they find that the stickiness of their blood is on the order of $4\frac{1}{5}$ times stickier than normal. Almost universally, doctors will prescribe a low-saturated-fat diet for these patients and explain to them that saturated fats are responsible for the formation of blood clots like the one that caused their problem.

This is only partially true, however. Some of the long-chain saturated fatty acids do increase the sticky qualities of blood. What many doctors fail to acknowledge, however, is that the polyunsaturated fats have the same effect. In fact, all dietary fats, with the important exception of omega-3 fats and medium-chain triglyceride (MCT) fats, promote blood stickiness.

MCTs, as found in coconut oil, do not have any effect on blood stickiness at all because MCTs are used up immediately for energy. Populations who consume the most coconut oil have the lowest percentage of heart disease and stroke related to blood stickiness factors and clotting disorders.

Atherosclerosis Facts

The interesting thing about atherosclerosis, or hardening of the arteries, is that almost no one seems to really understand how it occurs or, indeed, what it is. But if you ask someone to explain the disease to you, he or she will inevitably tell you, as sure as the sun rises in the east, that atherosclerosis occurs when arteries become clogged because of too much cholesterol in the blood. People reason that this must be the case. Otherwise, why would their doctors have prescribed medications to lower cholesterol? It all makes perfect sense—doesn't it?

Unfortunately, this idea is completely wrong. As previously mentioned, cholesterol does not circulate in the blood looking for a place to stick around and do damage to arterial walls. In fact, cholesterol is not even a necessary component of arterial plaque. You didn't know that? Maybe your doctor doesn't know that either.

The main component of arterial plaque is—drum roll, please—protein. Arterial plaques are made of protein in the form of scar tissue. But why on earth would there be scar tissue in your arteries? Ah well … that gets back to the earlier discussion about how cholesterol acts as a patch to help mend injuries. Our arteries sustain lots of injuries. Some of them are due to wear and tear brought on by high blood pressure. Other culprits include viruses, bacteria, free radicals, and toxins that circulate in the blood. For as long as these bad actors remain in the blood, they are wreaking havoc on your arterial walls. They cause injury, and in response to the inflammation they cause, your arteries develop tough scar tissue that begins the process of hardening arterial walls.

As time goes on, blood platelets encounter these injured sites, and as explained in the previous section, they react to the injury by becoming sticky and forming a clot to cover the injury and allow it to heal. In response to the formation of the blood clot, the artery wall releases protein growth factors. These, in turn, stimulate the growth of muscle in the arterial walls that reinforces and strengthens the injured artery. Over time a complex aggregate of tissue made up of platelets, minerals, protein, cholesterol, and triglycerides is laid down inside of the artery wall itself, not on the interior of the blood vessel's canal as is often thought. It is the mineral deposits and scar tissue laid down within the structure of the artery, in response to injury, that accounts for the hardening known as atherosclerosis.

Chronic Inflammatory Risk

There are many known risk factors for heart disease, but risk factors do not necessarily result in heart disease. For instance, cigarette smoking is a risk factor associated with heart disease. But if cigarette smoking were responsible, everyone who smokes would develop heart disease, and people who don't smoke would not. This is not the case. To the contrary, there are many people dying of heart disease who have few of the commonly associated risk factors. One extremely interesting idea regarding the progression of coronary artery disease has to do with chronic inflammation.

Based on the work of two-time Nobel Prize laureate Dr. Linus Pauling, it has been proposed that coronary artery disease is the result of chronic inflammation due to low-grade, chronic scurvy. Scurvy is a disease of malnutrition that, if acute and left untreated with sufficient amounts of vitamin C, results in death.

The Vitamin C Connection

Vitamin C, for most creatures, is not a vitamin at all but a hormone. Most animals are able to synthesize all the vitamin C they need, and the amount they have circulating in their systems varies profoundly according to the severity of inflammatory stressors they are experiencing at any given time. People, high-order primates, and guinea pigs, however, have somehow lost the ability to synthesize vitamin C. Humans must get vitamin C in their diets in sufficient quantities or they will die.

It has long been known, too, that human arteries weaken without the support provided by the presence of sufficient vitamin C. The plaques that form due to injury in arteries begin as soft atherosclerotic plaques known as atheromas. Dr. Pauling and his associates were the first to theorize that these plaques served to strengthen arteries because they seemed to appear most often where the blood pressure is highest.

Fortunately, atheromas in the tiny arteries in the retina of the eye can be seen by eye doctors, who have used them as markers for various disease processes. Until recently, however, it was thought that atheromas were irreversible. One doctor of ophthalmology in the United Kingdom, however, accidentally discovered that they are reversible.

Dr. Sydney Bush was looking for a way to prevent eye infections in patients who wore contact lenses. He instructed his patients to take large doses of supplementary vitamin C as a prophylactic because of the vitamin's antimicrobial and anti-inflammatory properties. As he followed these patients, he discovered that those patients who previously had atheromas in the retina no longer had them. They had disappeared.

This borders on a controversial issue regarding whether atherosclerosis is reversible with the sufficient administration of vitamin C. But what it does show is that coronary artery disease is due, at least in part, to repeated injury of arterial walls—some of which is caused by inflammation-causing viruses and bacteria—and that when the offenders and inflammation are removed, arteries begin to heal.

Disabling Persistent Chronic Infection

Most researchers are not yet ready to say that coronary heart disease is caused by infection—even though many cases of cardiomyopathy and endocarditis certainly are. Dentists, for example, will not clean the teeth of a person who has been diagnosed with mitral valve prolapse without first administering a prophylactic dose of antibiotics to prevent bacteria in the mouth from migrating to the heart and causing damage there.

Unfortunately, antibiotics are completely innocuous to viral agents. Viruses are completely unaffected by them. Some viruses persist, too, even after they seem to have run their course. Herpes zoster is a case in point. The herpes virus, which causes chicken pox, persists in the body indefinitely. It may reemerge as a painful case of shingles at some point, or it may lie undetectable for many years, but it lives on in the body, triggering immune responses that contribute to chronic stress for the immune system. When such viral agents enter the bloodstream, they can attach to arterial walls and cause low-grade chronic infections that cause further damage and lead to atherosclerosis.

While vitamin C and antibiotics may be of some help in disabling certain pathogens, there is a known substance that disables viruses, too. The medium-chain fatty acids in coconut oil destroy lipid-encapsulated viruses by dissolving their envelopes. At the same time, MCTs also disrupt a virus's ability to replicate itself. So MCTs work simultaneously on two fronts to reduce the load of bacteria, viruses, yeast, and fungi that would do harm to our tissues. At the same time, the anti-inflammatory properties of coconut oil work to calm and normalize inflamed tissue so that it can regain its normal function.

Oral Hygiene and Heart Disease

It may be difficult to imagine, but the condition of your mouth can seriously affect the health of the rest of your body. As previously mentioned, dentists have known this for years. They will not clean teeth in a person who has certain heart conditions without first administering antibiotic therapy. Some cancers even come under suspicion when certain types of bacteria are present in the mouth.

By the same token, the condition of the mouth is a mirror of the body's general health. People have always innately known this. Farmers examine the mouths of livestock before they seriously consider buying. People are attracted to others who have bright white, healthy smiles and a full set of straight teeth. In dentistry, an old idea known as the *focal infection theory* explains this. This theory states that an oral infection influences the health of the entire organism. Before modern dental techniques were developed, dentists would pull an infected tooth to prevent the infection from spreading to other parts of the body. Modern studies have borne out the fact that this old-fashioned notion was correct. Various investigations have shown that poor oral health is associated with kidney disease, diabetes, ulcers, heart disease, stroke, and atherosclerosis.

At the root of this is the oral environment. Dr. Bruce Fife describes the inside of our mouths as being like a tropical rain forest—this is a very astute observation. Inside our mouths live millions of bacteria, viruses, protozoa and yeasts, and dead cell debris of all kinds. The bacteria alone number more than 600 different kinds and total in the tens of millions. In his book *Oil Pulling Therapy*, Dr. Fife explains how coconut oil can be used in an ancient oral hygiene practice from Ayurvedic medicine that is astonishingly effective at removing bacteria and other pathogens from our mouths—pathogens that might otherwise go on to cause heart disease and many other maladies throughout the body. In the same way that coconut oil protects the skin of people from pathogens endemic to tropical environs, it can protect our mouths, too.

While Dr. Fife explains that any edible oil might be effective in removing bacteria, coconut oil—with its special antibacterial and antiviral properties—has the potential of doing a much more thorough job. Claims of warts falling off, remission of arthritic conditions, the resolution of fibromyalgia, and much, much more have been reported using this technique. If it's effective in resolving so many matters in the body, it's likely to be good for the cardiovascular system, too. To try oil pulling for yourself, see the recipe "Coconut Oil as a Mouthwash" in Chapter 18. Dr. Fife recommends repeating the procedure twice per day.

Industry, Politics, and Heart Disease

Unfortunately for the public, medicine and pharmaceuticals are big business. Coconut oil is an inexpensive and easily obtained natural product. Since there is no money to be made in conducting research or promoting a natural product that cannot be patented, coconut oil has largely been ignored by these two industries. Lipid scientists, clinicians, and others who research and report on the health benefits of coconut oil face a daunting battle in doing so because there is no funding available. At the same time, many prejudices against tropical oils still exist, leading to discredited research, discounted findings, and disregard for long-standing proofs.

The manufactured vegetable oil industry, too, has played a role in suppressing the truth about the health benefits of coconut oil—even while it was known as early as the 1950s that soybean oil caused health problems and weight gain. The manufactured oil industry is so powerful that to publish an unfavorable report on the dangers of hydrogenated oil is potentially career ending. The book *What Your Doctor Won't Tell You* by Jane Heimlich exposes just such a case, in which one researcher was no longer able to find funding for her work.

As reported by Dr. Mary Enig in her presentation to the Asian Pacific Coconut Community on its 36th anniversary, "Some of the food oil industry (especially those connected with the American Soybean Association [ASA]) and some of the consumer activists (especially the Center for Science in the Public Interest [CSPI] and also the American Heart Savers Association) further eroded the status of natural fats when they sponsored the major anti-saturated fat, anti-tropical oils campaign in the late 1980s."

In reality, the coconut industry has endured over 30 years of abusive rhetoric from groups like CSPI, the American Soybean Association, and others in the manufactured edible oil industry, and from those in the media and in the medical and scientific communities who have blindly repeated and promoted the misinformation propounded by those groups.

In August 1986, CSPI issued a news release criticizing what it called "Deceptive Vegetable Oil Labeling: Saturated Fat Without the Facts," that referred to "palm, coconut, and palm kernel oil" as "rich in artery-clogging saturated fat." At the same time, it announced that it was petitioning the U.S. Food and Drug Administration to disallow the labeling of foods as having "100 percent vegetable short-ening" if they contained tropical oils. In the same petition, CSPI further requested mandatory labeling of coconut, palm, and palm kernel oils as "a saturated fat" any time these ingredients appeared on food labels.

In 1988, CSPI published a booklet called "Saturated Fat Attack." It contained lists of processed foods CSPI found in Washington, D.C., supermarkets, and used those lists to develop their campaign against the saturated fats (tropical oils) contained in those products. Section III of the booklet was titled "Those Troublesome Tropical Oils," and it further encouraged pejorative labeling of tropical oils.

According to Dr. Enig, "There were lots of substantive mistakes in the booklet, including errors in the description of the biochemistry of fats and oils and completely erroneous statements about the fat and oil composition of many of the products." Because of the results brought by these and subsequent campaigns, it is obvious that industry holds some sway in government. The manufactured oil industry and related groups have been able to convolute truth and sway opinions of the various watchdogs of our health. Consequently, various authorities in health and nutrition have come out against coconut oil. In some cases, these authorities have had enough influence to convince folks in the coconut-growing regions of the world that consuming coconut oil causes heart disease.

In India, when government officials began to believe the manufactured oil industry's line and the people of India switched to eating margarines and other vegetable oils, the rate of heart disease tripled in only a few years. Obviously, coconut oil was not the cause of the tragic and dramatic increase in heart disease, and since then, Indian researchers have begun recommending a return to the traditional uses of coconut oil in the diet.

The Least You Need to Know

- Reducing consumption of naturally saturated fat does not reduce serum cholesterol. The types and levels of cholesterol in your blood are more dependent on your body's response to inflammation caused by a variety of other factors, including toxins, viral and bacterial invaders, and inadequate nutrition.

- Arterial plaques are primarily made up of protein in the form of scar tissue, and 74 percent of fat in these plaques are unsaturated fats.

- Medium-chain fatty acids, like those found in coconut oil, and omega-3 fats are the only fats that do not contribute to an increase in blood stickiness associated with clotting, which results in heart attacks and ischemic strokes.
- Chronic inflammation is the greatest risk factor for cardio-vascular disease, and oral hygiene has a great impact on the level of inflammation within the body.
- The pharmaceutical industry and the modern vegetable oil industry have no financial incentive for researching or accurately reporting on coconut oil, and the vegetable oil industry has worked to mislead and negatively influence government and health authorities' opinions of coconut oil to the public's detriment.

Other Health Benefits of Coconut Oil

In This Chapter

- Stopping the cravings
- Living pain free with energy to spare
- Maintaining healthy bundles of joy

From type 2 diabetes to cradle cap, from irritable bowel syndrome to cracked nipples, coconut oil seems to have countless healthful applications. Whether used in the diet or applied to the skin, the healthy medium-chain fatty acids in coconut oil work to improve immunity, disable viruses and bacteria, and protect against yeast infection and protozoa infestation.

This chapter explores how the lauric, capric, and caprylic acids in coconut can help diabetics; aid those plagued by irritable bowel syndrome, Crohn's disease, fibromyalgia, and chronic fatigue; and be of tremendous benefit in the infant care and feeding.

Type 2 Diabetes

Coconut oil, especially when coupled with a low-carbohydrate diet, has many benefits for the diabetic. Coconut oil is known to satiate hunger, combat yeast infection (to which diabetics are prone), and increase metabolism while providing ketones for energy (bypassing the need for glucose and eliminating spikes and crashes in blood-sugar and insulin levels).

> **TO YOUR HEALTH!**
>
> "Indeed virgin coconut oil has a substantial effect on blood-sugar levels. My wife and daughter [who both have type 2 diabetes] measure their blood sugar levels at least three times a day. When they eat the wrong foods and their blood-sugar levels get to 80–100 points above normal, they don't take extra medication; they take 2–3 tablespoons of coconut oil directly from the bottle. Within a half hour their blood sugar levels will come back to normal." ~Ed
>
> —Brian and Marianita Shilhavy, *Virgin Coconut Oil*

Diabetes is rare in populations that consume most of their calories in the form of coconut oil's saturated fats. In 1998, a study conducted in India found that when Indians switched from eating their traditional fats like coconut oil and ghee and started using polyunsaturated fats, their rates of diabetes skyrocketed. Other population studies, like those conducted in the South Pacific, have shown that when the traditional diet, including large quantities of coconut oil, transitioned to foods containing polyunsaturated fats, there was a direct correlation in the increase of diabetes and other Western diseases.

Fibromyalgia and Chronic Fatigue Syndrome

Fibromyalgia and chronic fatigue syndrome (CFS) are associated with the Epstein-Barr virus. Epstein-Barr is one of the lipid-encapsulated viruses that coconut oil is able to disrupt and destroy by dissolving the virus's fatty envelope. This envelope is a protective covering—like a skin or a shell—that encases the virus's protein shell (known as a capsid) and its genetic material.

> **TO YOUR HEALTH!**
>
> "I, too, have had very painful fibromyalgia for the past 15 years or so. I have been using the virgin coconut oil now for two months and have no pain at all. No pain!!! And I have a lot more energy. And my skin has never looked so good. For me, I call it my Miracle VCO [virgin coconut oil]." ~Danne
>
> —Brian and Marianita Shilhavy, *Virgin Coconut Oil*

There is another theory concerning CFS and fibromyalgia, though. Some alternative medicine practitioners believe that these diseases are really the result of poor thyroid function. If this is the case, as discussed in Chapter 10, coconut oil—especially in conjunction with a healthy, low-carbohydrate diet—can support the thyroid and bring relief, too.

Crohn's Disease

Ever since Alka-Seltzer's TV advertisements of the late 1960s and early 1970s proclaimed, "I can't believe I ate the whole thing!" and "*Mama mia*, that's a spicy meatball!" commercials have poked fun at stomach upsets. But digestive disorders are no laughing matter. Many such disorders are the cause of serious pain, problems of malabsorption, and near-complete disruption of normal life. Crohn's disease is one of these.

Many people have reported significant relief from the symptoms of Crohn's disease after adding coconut oil to their diets. In their book, *The People's Pharmacy Guide to Home and Herbal Remedies*, pharmacist Joe Graedon and his wife Dr. Teresa Graedon shared a letter that told the tale of an incredible experience involving Crohn's disease, chronic diarrhea, and coconut macaroons.

As the story goes, an unfortunate man had suffered with the chronic pain and diarrhea that accompanies Crohn's disease for 40 years. He said that sometimes Lomotil would help a little, but it didn't give him any real relief. He went on to write that since he had bought a box of coconut macaroons a couple of months earlier and had begun eating two per day, his diarrhea stopped—and that if he ate more than two he would become constipated. Talk about a new lease on life!

The same man also told of his brother-in-law's friend who had chronic diarrhea as a result of a cancer surgery. When the men told him about how macaroons had cleared up Crohn's disease diarrhea, the cancer patient decided it couldn't hurt him to give macaroons a try. Almost incredibly, coconut macaroons did the trick for this cancer patient as well.

When the Graedons published this letter, it set off a coconut macaroon craze in the coconut oil forums, and since then a tremendous number of people have reported similar good results.

Irritable Bowel Syndrome (IBS)

According to WebMD, irritable bowel syndrome (IBS) affects up to 55 million Americans—mostly women—and its cause is unknown. The debilitating symptoms of IBS include diarrhea, constipation, and abdominal cramping, and while there is no known cure, diet and lifestyle changes can help.

> **TO YOUR HEALTH!**
>
> "I've been using coconut oil about a month now, 2 teaspoons per day. Mix it in anything possible or just throw it on top of pizza slices. I have IBS and am a compulsive overeater. Within a short time of taking it, I realized I was no longer wanting food. In the past month I have lost 5 pounds and just as many inches. Instead of being a computer potato, I am up and about doing things … I just have so much energy. The biggest change is the IBS. Instead of the runs, now I almost need laxatives. *laughing* It's been since my early 20s that I've felt this way … I'm 42 now. Coconut oil is fantastic!!!" ~Net B.
>
> —Brian and Marianita Shilhavy, *Virgin Coconut Oil*

It seems, however, that some cases of IBS may be caused by a parasite known as giardia. An expert in diseases of the gastrointestinal tract, Dr. Leo Galland, found that half of the 200 patients with IBS symptoms he examined were infected with giardia.

Coconut oil is able to provide protection against many parasites, including giardia. Like many bacteria and viruses, some protozoa like giardia cannot survive exposure to coconut oil's medium-chain fatty acids.

Dr. Bruce Fife relates that, in India, coconut oil has been used in the removal of tapeworms and that feeding animals ground coconut has been a successful remedy for pets' intestinal parasites as well. Tapeworms, lice, yeast, fungi, viruses, bacteria, and protozoa, like giardia, can all be eliminated or held in check by the liberal use of coconut oil.

Coconut Oil in Infant Care and Feeding

Just as in the care of the elderly demented (see Chapter 9), coconut oil is extremely useful in infant care and feeding. Dr. Fife describes in his book, *The Coconut Oil Miracle,* how Polynesian mothers traditionally slathered their newborns with coconut oil daily as a nourishing barrier against their harsh tropical environment and that they continued to do so daily until the children were old enough to do so themselves.

But beyond skin protection, there is much more coconut oil can do. Because of its high lauric acid content, coconut oil is an excellent ingredient to add to baby's first foods.

Lauric Acid in Mother's Milk

Lauric acid is an important component of mother's milk, and it is integral to the synthesis of monolaurin, which is important to healthy immune function. For babies, it is an essential fatty acid. So if a baby is not being breast-fed, it becomes all the more important for lauric acid to be part of the baby's infant formula and the other foods in his or her diet.

Adding coconut oil to a baby's foods and beverages is an effortless way of accomplishing this. Just a half-teaspoon added to a bottle of warm infant formula will provide an abundance of lauric acid over the course of a day.

Later, when children begin eating solid foods like cereals and mashed vegetables, stirring a little coconut oil into these, using your baby's spoon size as a guide, provides more of the health-giving properties of coconut oil as your child progresses toward weaning.

Diaper Rash, Thrush, and (Ouch!) Cracked Nipples

Another important component of coconut oil is its capric and caprylic acid content. Both of these medium-chain fatty acids provide protection against yeast infection.

In babies, yeast infection often presents as a red, raised, bumpy diaper rash that can be difficult to treat. Coconut oil applied to the diaper area after every washing and diaper change helps to prevent yeast from colonizing baby's delicate skin. If a little rash does begin to develop, fresh air, a little sunshine, and coconut oil will take care of it in no time at all.

Yeast is present on our skin surfaces and does not usually cause an infection unless the skin is somehow damaged. But babies can pick up yeast in the course of feeding (either from a bottle or in breast-feeding), and yeast can colonize your baby's mouth, too. This painful infection, known as thrush, can make it difficult for the baby to feed. The capric and caprylic acids in coconut oil make it difficult for yeast to find a comfortable environment in the baby's mouth. Furthermore, since the yeast do not overgrow in your baby's mouth, there will be fewer to move on to his or her digestive tract and, ultimately, be excreted into his diaper—another method of diaper rash avoidance!

Finally, there is the painful possibility of cracked nipples. If you breastfeed your child, it is likely that at some point your nipples will become sore, inflamed, or even cracked. Unfortunately, these sorts of complications have caused many women to stop breastfeeding earlier than they'd planned. Using coconut oil on nipples before and after feeding is soothing to Mom. Moreover, coconut oil provides antimicrobial benefits that prevent irritated nipples from progressing to infected nipples and precipitating *mastitis!*

DEFINITION

Mastitis is a breast infection typically caused by *Staphylococcus aureus,* a common bacteria found on skin. The bacteria enter through an injury or crack in the skin, usually on the nipple. The infection takes place in the fatty tissue of the breast and causes painful swelling and lumps in the infected breast's tissue.

An added benefit of applying coconut oil to the nipples when breast-feeding is that the baby also receives an application in his mouth! This is a further preventative against oral thrush or yeast infection.

Baby Boys

Many parents choose to have their baby boys circumcised, either out of religious convictions, a concern for hygiene, or social concerns. But circumcision is not a procedure on the order of clipping toenails! The circumcised child will be extremely sensitive and experience some degree of pain for many days. Coconut oil applied to the circumcised area of the penis will prevent this delicate tissue from adhering to the diaper, which can cause a painful tear. Coconut oil also helps keep the delicate tissue moisturized and comfortable while providing a natural barrier to bacteria, diaper soils, and yeast.

Navel Care

The area around the umbilicus is another area that is prone to bacterial or yeast infection—especially in newborns. Sometimes the umbilical stump takes longer than usual to fall off, and this is a further invitation to infection. The antibacterial properties found in coconut oil keep opportunistic bacteria and yeast at bay while the navel area heals. It also provides a barrier to the moisture that comes from being covered in a warm diaper on hot days and the urine and ammonia that can accumulate in a diaper overnight.

Cradle Cap

Finally, though not a health concern, many babies develop cradle cap. Parents who worry about this accumulation of sebum on the scalp of their newborns will find that it is easily removed with an application of coconut oil.

Simply apply a generous dab of coconut oil to the hair and scalp of your baby. Gently massage it in well and allow the oil to remain for several hours or overnight. In the morning, the cradle cap should be very easily removed with gentle washing and by combing through the hair with a fine-toothed baby's comb.

The Least You Need to Know

- Coconut oil works to satiate hunger and to end overeating and sugar cravings. It also helps balance blood-sugar and insulin levels in the diabetic. Diabetes is rarely found in populations that traditionally consume lots of coconut.

- Many people have reported relief from the pain and fatigue of fibromyalgia and chronic fatigue syndrome after adding coconut oil to their diets.

- IBS and Crohn's disease sufferers find surprising relief from painful cramping, embarrassing gas, and debilitating diarrhea after consuming coconut macaroons.

- Coconut oil's medium-chain fatty acids nourish a baby's immature immune system and provide protection to delicate skin against opportunistic bacteria and yeast—to both the baby and mother.

Coconut Oil Recipes

When Westerners think about coconut recipes, usually the first thing that comes to mind is something along the lines of coconut cream pie. While coconut cream pie is a delightful dessert, to think that dessert is where coconut begins and ends does no justice to the incredible versatility of coconut and coconut oil.

In Part 4, we introduce delicious recipes that explore coconut cuisine straight from the tropical shores of Tahiti, India, Hawaii, and Samoa. Then we delve into the incredibly rich possibilities for coconut in exciting soups, curries, and condiments—giving a special nod to Thailand and Brazil. As far as sweets and treats go, we suggest delightful coconut recipes that fit the high standards of dementia patients and acknowledge the time constraints of caregivers' needs.

Because coconut oil nourishes the body from the outside, too, the final chapter in Part 4 offers recipes for natural homemade hygiene, hair, and skin-care products.

Main Dishes and Sides

In This Chapter

- Embracing world cuisines
- Exploring protein possibilities
- Using side dishes to enhance your meal

By adding coconut oil and other coconut products to your cooking repertoire, you instantly open the door to a fascinating adventure into the realm of world cuisines. From Hawaii to India and from South America to the Middle East, coconut is used in the most exciting and delectable ways.

These recipes are just a starting point in your world tour and include healthy examples of main-dish meals using each of the popular main proteins—poultry, pork, red meat, and a variety of seafood. To accompany your entrées, lovely sides that go with almost anything have also been included—fragrant spiced rice dishes, vegetable casseroles, a fun and easy bread, and a hearty vegetable-based dipping sauce.

Set your sails for a new destination. The whirlwind journey bound for new taste sensations and healthier meals begins right here.

Luau Chicken

Chicken in coconut milk is a standard native-Hawaiian luau dish with flavors non-natives find unusual. In this version, the traditional taro leaves are replaced with the comforting and familiar flavor of fresh spinach.

Yielid:	Prep time:	Cook time:	Serving size:
8 pieces chicken	10 minutes	40 minutes	2 pieces chicken

Each serving has:			
109 g carbohydrate	50.9 g fat	9.7 g fiber	75.8 g protein
27.75 g coconut oil = 1.85 TB.			

2 lb. fresh spinach	1 (3-lb.) fryer chicken, cut into 8 portions and patted dry
1 cup cornstarch	¼ cup coconut oil
1 TB. coarse salt	1 cup chicken broth
1 TB. garlic powder	3 cups coconut milk
1 TB. onion powder	
1 tsp. freshly ground black pepper	

1. Wash spinach and remove stems. Stack leaves and roughly chop in half.

2. Combine cornstarch, salt, garlic powder, onion powder, and black pepper in a plastic zipper bag. Place chicken pieces, one or two at a time, in the bag and shake thoroughly to coat. Set aside.

3. Heat coconut oil in a large skillet that has a lid. When oil is hot, sauté chicken pieces, uncovered, until golden brown on all sides.

4. Add chicken broth to the skillet and bring to a simmer. Cover the skillet and continue cooking about 30 minutes or until chicken is tender.

5. Taste broth for seasoning and adjust if necessary. Keep the skillet warm over very low heat to maintain temperature.

6. In a separate large skillet, sauté spinach in only the water that remains on the leaves. When wilted and tender, add 2 cups coconut milk. Bring to a simmer and continue to cook for 1 minute more.

7. Arrange chicken portions in the center of a large, deep platter or casserole. Surround chicken with prepared spinach and coconut milk.

8. Heat remaining 1 cup coconut milk but do not allow it to boil. Pour coconut milk over chicken and spinach. Serve hot.

TO YOUR HEALTH!

If you can locate a source of fresh taro leaves, you may want to give them a try. Taro leaves are a good source of niacin, vitamin B_6, and phosphorus and are an excellent source of fiber, thiamin, riboflavin, folate, calcium, iron, magnesium, potassium, copper, manganese, and vitamins A, C, E, and K.

Want more? Taro leaves also are a complete protein source—something rarely found in vegetables—providing adequate proportions of all nine essential amino acids!

Chicken Keo Keo

Ginger and sherry–marinated chicken define the flavor of this elegant Hawaiian dish that is traditionally served inside a flavorful young, fresh coconut.

Yield:	Prep time:	Cook time:	Serving size:
9 cups	1 hour (marinating time)	30 minutes	1½ cups

Each serving has:			
25 g carbohydrate	28.3 g fat	5.5 g fiber	55.2 g protein
7.5 g coconut oil = .5 TB. (more if served in a fresh coconut)			

6 boneless, skinless chicken breasts, cubed

½ cup light soy sauce

1 TB. granulated sugar

3 tsp. sherry

2 slices (¼ in. thick) ginger root, minced

3 TB. coconut oil

2 garlic cloves, minced

3 ribs bok choy, sliced diagonally ⅛ in. thick

½ lb. fresh mushrooms, sliced

½ lb. green peas, fresh or frozen

1 quart chicken broth

½ tsp. salt

Dash freshly ground black pepper

3 TB. cornstarch mixed into ¼ cup water

1 (5-oz.) can bamboo shoots, rinsed and drained

1 (5-oz.) can water chestnuts, rinsed, drained, and diced

¼ lb. almonds, toasted

1. Combine cubed chicken, light soy sauce, sugar, sherry, and ginger root in a nonmetallic bowl. Toss to coat chicken and allow to marinate, covered, for 1 hour at room temperature.

2. Reserving marinade, drain chicken and set aside on paper towels.

3. In a large skillet over medium heat, heat coconut oil and sauté garlic and cubed chicken until chicken browns. Remove chicken to a bowl and set aside.

4. Adding more oil to the skillet if necessary, sauté bok choy along with mushrooms for 3 minutes.

5. Add green peas and cook for 2 minutes more.

6. Stir in chicken broth and marinade and bring to a boil. Reduce heat and allow sauce to simmer for 5 minutes more.

7. Return chicken to the skillet and add salt and black pepper. Simmer for 5 minutes.

8. Stir in cornstarch slurry and continue cooking until sauce has thickened.

9. Stir in bamboo shoots and water chestnuts, cover, and remove from heat.

10. Serve hot in coconut shell halves, garnished with toasted almonds.

> **TROPICAL TIP**
>
> Economically minded cooks can reuse coconut shell bowls by hand-washing and rinsing them well. Air dry shells and store in zipper bags in the freezer until ready to use again.

Orange Coconut Chicken

Orange, coconut, and cinnamon flavor this interesting island-style chicken dish.

Yield:	Prep time:	Cook time:	Serving size:
8 pieces chicken	1 hour	1 hour	2 pieces chicken

Each serving has:			
38.4 g carbohydrate	20.8 g fat	1.2 g fiber	100.8 g protein
12.7 g coconut oil = .85 TB.			

1 (3-lb.) fryer chicken, cut into 8 serving pieces	½ tsp. cinnamon, ground
3 TB. soy sauce	1 slice (¼ in. thick) ginger root, minced
3 TB. cornstarch	½ cup white seedless raisins
3 TB. coconut oil (RBD or expeller pressed is best)	1 tsp. salt
2 cups orange juice	Hot cooked rice
2 TB. brown sugar	Flaked coconut, toasted

1. Rinse and pat chicken dry. Sprinkle with soy sauce and then cornstarch. Massage around with your hands to coat well. Set aside for 1 hour.

2. Reserving soy sauce, drain chicken.

3. In a large skillet, heat coconut oil and brown chicken on all sides. Remove chicken and set aside.

4. Add orange juice and reserved soy sauce to pan juices in the skillet, scraping to deglaze the pan.

5. Add brown sugar, cinnamon, ginger root, white seedless raisins, and salt to the skillet and simmer for 45 minutes, covered.

6. Serve chicken pieces arranged on a bed of hot rice. Top with pan sauce and garnish with toasted coconut.

Roasted Coconut Chicken

The bright and warming flavors of orange and ginger, and the crispy cornflake crumb texture, make this roasted chicken dish great for special occasions.

Yield:	Prep time:	Cook time:	Serving size:
8 pieces chicken	2 hours (marinating time)	2 hours	1 or 2 pieces chicken

Each serving has:			
31.4 g carbohydrate	31.2 g fat	6.6 g fiber	73.2 g protein
22.2 g coconut oil = 1.5 TB.			

1 roasting chicken, cut into 8 serving pieces	½ tsp. garlic powder
1 small can frozen orange juice, defrosted	2 cups chicken broth
	1 tsp. lemon juice
½ tsp. salt	Freshly ground black pepper (optional)
2 slices (¼ in. thick) fresh ginger root, minced	2 TB. cornstarch mixed with ¼ cup water
½ cup cornflake crumbs	Parsley
1 bag shredded coconut	1 whole fresh orange, thinly sliced
2 large eggs, beaten	
1 TB. soy sauce	2 or 3 cups freshly cooked rice

1. Rinse chicken and pat dry.

2. Mix together orange juice, salt, and ginger root in a deep nonmetallic baking dish. Add chicken, turning to coat. Cover and marinate at room temperature for 2 hours, turning occasionally.

3. Reserving marinade, drain juices from chicken. Set marinade aside.

4. Mix cornflake crumbs with shredded coconut and spread on a baking sheet.

5. In a medium bowl, mix beaten eggs with soy sauce, garlic powder, and half of reserved marinade.

6. One piece at a time, dip chicken pieces into egg mixture and then roll in the coconut/cornflake mixture. Press cornflakes and coconut onto chicken if necessary.

7. Place each chicken piece onto a greased baking pan, skin-side up, and bake at 350°F for 1 to 1½ hours or until juices run clear. Remove chicken pieces to a serving platter, keep warm, and set aside.

8. Pour pan juices into a small saucepan and add remaining marinade, chicken broth, lemon juice, and black pepper (if using). Bring to a high simmer over medium heat.

9. Stir in the cornstarch slurry and cook while stirring until sauce thickens. Pour sauce into a gravy boat.

10. Serve chicken garnished with fresh parsley and thinly sliced oranges, accompanied by hot fresh rice topped with orange-chicken gravy.

TO YOUR HEALTH!

According to the National Institutes of Health, preliminary research suggests that eating garlic (*Allium sativum*) could slow the development of atherosclerosis, a hardening of the arteries that can lead to heart disease or stroke.

Molokai Roast Pork with Coconut–Peanut Butter Crust

Peanut butter and coconut–encrusted pork with top notes of orange and ginger is sure to be a hit!

Yield:	Prep time:	Cook time:	Serving size:
8 (12-ounce) slices	5 minutes	2½ to 3 hours	1 slice

Each serving has:			
4.9 g carbohydrate	21 g fat	2 g fiber	92.1 g protein
4.5 g coconut oil = .3 tablespoon			

6 lb. boneless pork loin roast

¼ cup peanut butter

¼ cup coconut cream concentrate

½ cup orange juice

¼ cup soy sauce

1 slice (¼ in. thick) ginger root, minced

Optional garnishes: pineapple chunks, sliced oranges or limes, or whole kumquats

1. Set pork loin roast on a roasting rack in a roaster pan with 2 inches of hot water in the bottom of the pan.

2. Roast for 2 hours at 300°F or until internal temperature registers 145°F.

3. In a small mixing bowl, combine peanut butter, coconut cream concentrate, orange juice, soy sauce, and ginger root.

4. Remove the pan from the oven and brush seasoning mixture over roast's surface.

5. Return roast to the oven and continue to baste frequently with peanut butter mixture until roast is fully coated and beautifully brown (about 30 to 45 minutes).

6. Remove roast to a serving platter and allow to rest 20 minutes before carving.

7. Serve garnished with a variety of fresh fruits such as pineapple chunks, sliced oranges or limes, or whole kumquats.

TROPICAL TIP

This recipe can be prepared on a grill over medium-hot coals using a rotisserie spit, too!

Filipino-Style Pork and Noodles (Pansit)

Lean pork and traditional Asian spices define this favorite noodle dish from the Philippines.

Yield:	Prep time:	Cook time:	Serving size:
6 generous soup bowls	20 minutes	50 minutes	1 soup bowl

Each serving has:			
46.9 g carbohydrate	19.3 g fat	3.4 g fiber	45.9 g protein
9 g coconut oil = .6 TB.			

3 TB. coconut oil

2 cloves garlic, minced

1 slice (¼ in. thick) ginger root, minced

1 medium onion, thinly sliced

2 ribs celery, thinly sliced

1 lb. pork stew meat

½ lb. chicken breast meat, cut into thin strips

3 TB. soy sauce

3 medium fresh tomatoes, sliced

1 TB. granulated sugar

½ lb. thin rice or egg noodles, cooked and drained

Optional garnishes: chopped raw peanuts, lemon slices, chopped green onions, sliced hard-boiled eggs

1. In a large skillet, heat coconut oil and sauté garlic, ginger root, onion, and celery until onion is golden brown. Remove vegetables from the pan and set aside.

2. Add more oil to the skillet if necessary and brown pork and chicken meat.

3. Add soy sauce, tomatoes, and sugar to meat. Return seasoning vegetables to the pan, combine well, and simmer over medium-low heat, covered, for about 45 minutes.

4. Place rice noodles in the pan and continue to cook until noodles are fully heated through.

5. Serve garnished with any combination of chopped raw peanuts, lemon slices, chopped green onions, and sliced hard-boiled eggs.

Variation: Substitute 1 pound of medium (40- to 50-count) shrimp for the pork and 4 cups thinly sliced cabbage for the tomatoes.

DEFINITION

Pansit (sometimes **pancit**) is the Filipino word for noodles, which happen to be very popular in Philippine cuisine. Philippine restaurants specializing in noodles are often referred to as *panciterias*—a term that melds Tagalog and Hispanic word origins.

Meatballs Bali

Toasted almonds, freshly chopped chives, green grapes, and shredded coconut add color and flavor to this sweet and sour dish.

Yield:	Prep time:	Cook time:	Serving size:
3 dozen meatballs	30 minutes	1 hour	6 meatballs

Each serving has:			
39.2 g carbohydrate	24.4 g fat	4 g fiber	52.4 g protein
5 g coconut oil = .33 TB.			

2 lb. ground beef

1½ tsp. salt

½ tsp. freshly ground black pepper

¼ cup dry breadcrumbs

¼ cup flaked coconut

3 cloves garlic, minced

1 tsp. paprika

1 small onion, grated, plus 1 small onion, finely chopped

2 large eggs, beaten with ¼ cup water

½ cup cornstarch

3 TB. coconut oil

1 slice (¼ in. thick) ginger root, minced

1 medium green bell pepper, seeded and sliced

1 medium red bell pepper, seeded and sliced

1 (13-oz.) can pineapple chunks

2 cups chicken broth

3 TB. soy sauce

¼ cup vinegar

3 TB. brown sugar

2 TB. honey

½ tsp. Chinese five-spice powder

Hot cooked rice

Toasted almonds

Fresh chives, chopped

1 cup shredded coconut

Green seedless grapes, halved

1. In a large mixing bowl, combine ground beef, 1 teaspoon salt, ¼ teaspoon black pepper, breadcrumbs, flaked coconut, 2 minced garlic cloves, paprika, grated onion, and beaten egg and water mixture.

2. Wet hands to thoroughly combine and form mixture into golf ball–size meatballs.

3. Lightly dredge meatballs in cornstarch and quickly brown balls in hot coconut oil in a large, heavy skillet— occasionally adding more oil as necessary.

4. As they finish, remove meatballs to paper towels to drain.

5. Carefully drain all but 2 tablespoons of oil from skillet and sauté remaining 1 minced garlic clove, ginger root, and chopped onion for 1 minute.

6. Add green bell pepper and red bell pepper and sauté until onion is translucent.

7. Reserving fruit, add pineapple juice and meatballs to the skillet and simmer for 10 minutes.

8. Add reserved pineapple, chicken broth, soy sauce, vinegar, brown sugar, honey, Chinese five-spice powder, remaining ½ teaspoon salt, and remaining ¼ tea-spoon black pepper to the skillet.

9. Bring sauce to a boil, reduce heat, and simmer for 5 minutes more.

10. Serve meatballs and sauce over hot, freshly cooked rice and garnished with almonds, chives, coconut, and grapes.

TROPICAL TIP

It is often easier, when preparing a large number of meatballs, to do so by placing them on a baking sheet and roasting them in a 375°F oven for 15 to 20 minutes, or until they have browned. Use oven-roasted meatballs immediately or store in the freezer in zipper bags until ready to use.

Beef or Lamb Madras

This popular meat dish from the cuisine of Southern India results in a wonderfully full-bodied, piquant blend of flavors that have come to be favorites around the world.

Yield:	Prep time:	Cook time:	Serving size:
12 cups	30 minutes	1½ hours	2 cups

Each serving has:			
58.6 g carbohydrate	26.4 g fat	3.1 g fiber	63.4 g protein
15 g coconut oil = 1 TB.			

6 TB. virgin coconut oil

2 medium onions, coarsely chopped

1-in. piece ginger root, peeled and coarsely chopped

4 cloves garlic, peeled and coarsely chopped

3 to 6 dried red chiles (These are hot! Use according to your taste.)

2 large cloves garlic, crushed and skins removed

2 fresh green chiles, sliced in half lengthwise

1 (14.5-oz.) can stewed tomatoes with juice

1 tsp. chili powder

1 tsp. coriander

3 tsp. ground cumin

1 tsp. ground turmeric

2½ lb. beef stew meat (or leg or shoulder of lamb), trimmed of fat and cut into 1½-in. cubes

¾ cup warm water

1¼ tsp. salt

1 tsp. garam masala

2 cups basmati rice, cooked

1. Put 3 tablespoons virgin coconut oil into a medium heavy skillet and sauté onions, ginger root, chopped garlic, and red chiles over medium heat until onions are soft. Set mixture aside and allow to cool.

2. In a heavy-bottomed Dutch oven, heat remaining 3 tablespoons oil and sauté crushed garlic and green chiles over medium heat until garlic just begins to lightly brown.

3. Add half of tomatoes and juice, chili powder, coriander, ground cumin, and ground turmeric to mixture. Stir and cook for a couple minutes more.

4. Adjust heat to low and continue to cook, stirring frequently, for about 10 more minutes to allow flavors to begin to meld.

5. Add beef stew meat to tomato mixture and readjust the heat to medium or medium-high until meat begins to brown.

6. Add warm water and bring the pot to a boil. Cover, reduce heat, and allow to simmer for 30 minutes.

7. Place remaining tomatoes and juice and sautéed onion mixture in a food processor and process. When mixture is smooth, add mixture and salt to meat.

8. Stir well and cover the pot. Allow it to continue simmering an additional 35 to 45 minutes.

10. When meat is tender, remove it from the heat and stir in garam masala.

11. Serve hot with freshly cooked basmati for a special Southern Indian treat.

TROPICAL TIP

Madras curries tend to be a bit spicier than other Indian curries, but it certainly is acceptable to vary the heat according to your diners' taste preferences. In fact, it is best for those who are unaccustomed to using hot chilies to go very lightly when first experimenting with curry dishes.

Marinated Fish in Coconut Cream (Ceviche)

Refreshing, brightly flavored *ceviches* are typically eaten at lunchtime or for brunch since the morning catch of fish will no longer be fresh enough for this dish by mid-afternoon.

Yield:	Prep time:	Serving size:	
4 cups	4 hours (marinating time)	1 cup	

Each serving has:			
11.1 g carbohydrate	12.2 g fat	3.3 g fiber	21.2 g protein
3.2 g coconut oil = .21 TB.			

1 tsp. sea salt	1 medium tomato, chopped
½ cup lime juice	1 clove garlic, crushed and minced
1 TB. *whey*	¾ cup coconut milk
1 lb. freshly caught whitefish, cleaned and cut into ½-in. cubes	1 head lettuce (Bibb lettuce works well)
1 bunch green onions, chopped	1 TB. sesame seeds, toasted

1. In a medium glass or ceramic mixing bowl, combine sea salt, lime juice, and whey.

2. Stir cubed whitefish into marinade to coat well, cover, and place in the refrigerator for at least 4 hours.

3. Using a colander, drain marinade away from fish.

4. Return fish to bowl and toss in green onions, tomato, and garlic.

5. Stir in coconut milk.

6. Place a bed of lettuce leaves on each of 4 chilled plates and mound 1 cup fish mixture on top.

7. Garnish with sesame seeds and serve immediately.

Ceviches are popular raw, marinated fish dishes in Asia, Latin America, Hawaii, and Scandinavia. The process of marinating the fish in an acidic solution of lime juice, lemon juice, or whey effectively kills any parasites or other pathogens that may have been present.

Whey is the liquid milk serum that remains after milk has been curdled and strained, such as in cheese or yogurt making. To make your own whey, line a sieve with a layer of cheesecloth and place it over a bowl. Pour a carton of plain yogurt onto the cheesecloth and allow it to stand at room temperature for several hours. The whey will separate from the yogurt and can be stored, refrigerated, in a glass jar for up to six months. The yogurt "cheese" makes a yummy spread for bagels!

Tahitian Fish (Poisson Cru)

This chilled fish appetizer is a brightly flavored lemon-coconut ceviche.

Yield:	Prep time:	Serving size:	
5 cups	3 hours (marinating time)	½ cup	

Each serving has:			
3 g carbohydrate	.7 g fat	0 g fiber	12.2 g protein
2.6 g coconut oil = .17 TB.			

1½ lb. freshly caught firm whitefish	3 TB. grated onion
1 tsp. coarse salt	1½ cups canned coconut milk
Fresh juice of 6 lemons	Cooked rice (at room temperature)

1. Cut whitefish into cubes. Place in a glass bowl and season with salt, lemon juice, and onion.

2. Cover and refrigerate overnight, turning fish occasionally.

3. Drain fish, add coconut milk, and chill for 2 to 3 hours more.

4. Serve on a bed of rice on a small salad plate as a first course.

Island Fish in Shrimp Sauce

Fish steaks topped with a richly flavorful, elegant shrimp sauce make a hearty meal.

Yield:	Prep time:	Serving size:
6 steaks	1 hour (marinating time)	1 steak

Each serving has:			
9 g carbohydrate	17.9 g fat	0 g fiber	43.5 g protein
40 g coconut oil = 2.7 TB.			

3 lb. mahi-mahi, cod steak, or swordfish, cut ¾ in. thick

3 TB. lemon juice

¼ cup butter, melted

½ tsp. salt

⅛ tsp. freshly ground black pepper

1 can cream of shrimp soup

½ cup Herbed Mayonnaise (see recipe in Chapter 16)

½ cup raw small (50- to 60-count) salad shrimp

2 fresh green onions (scallions), sliced

1. Rinse, dry, and cut fish into six portions.

2. Arrange portions in an ovenproof baking dish.

3. Sprinkle with lemon juice and allow to marinate in the refrigerator for 1 hour.

4. Drain fish, pour melted butter over fish, and season with salt and black pepper.

5. Broil fish for 10 minutes, about 4 inches from the flame.

6. Baste fish with butter and juices from the pan. Set aside to cool.

7. In a small bowl, mix cream of shrimp soup and Herbed Mayonnaise together, combining thoroughly. Top each fish portion with mixture, evenly divided.

8. Return fish to the oven and bake at 350°F until fish flakes, about 25 minutes.

9. Top with shrimp and bake only until shrimp turn pink.

10. Serve hot, garnished with fresh green onions.

> **TROPICAL TIP**
>
> Nothing can really compare with freshly caught mahi-mahi, but frozen mahi-mahi is also very good. If you can't find mahi-mahi though, any firm-fleshed fish can be substituted for it when baking, broiling, or pan-frying.

Samoan-Style Dolphinfish (Mahi-Mahi) in Coconut Milk

This is a versatile recipe that makes the unique flavor of your mahi-mahi really shine.

Yield:	Prep time:	Cook time:	Serving size:
2 pounds fish with sauce	10 minutes	20 minutes	10 ounces fish with sauce
Each serving has:			
8.4 g carbohydrate	30.1 g fat	1.9 g fiber	38.3 g protein
5.7 g coconut oil = .38 TB.			

2 lb. mahi-mahi	5 TB. butter (ghee, if available)
1 tsp. salt	2 cups coconut milk
²⁄₃ cup all-purpose flour	

1. Season mahi-mahi with salt and dredge in all-purpose flour.

2. Melt butter in a large skillet over medium-high heat and quickly sauté fish until golden brown.

3. Add coconut milk and simmer, covered, for 10 minutes.

4. Remove fish and sauce to a deep serving platter.

5. Cut fish into 6 equal portions and serve immediately topped with a generous amount of coconut sauce.

Variation: Substitute flounder for the mahi-mahi and finish, uncovered, in a 350°F oven for 15 minutes.

TROPICAL TIP

In the islands of Polynesia, squid is a favorite seafood and is traditionally prepared in the manner described here.

Tahitian Seafood Mélange

Tropical herbs and spices come together with tart apple, sumptuous lobster, shrimp, and crab.

Yield:	Prep time:	Cook time:	Serving size:
10 cups	20 minutes	20 minutes	1½ cups

Each serving has:			
12.7 g carbohydrate	37.9 g fat	2.9 g fiber	49.4 g protein
5.6 g coconut oil = .38 TB.			

¼ lb. (4 TB. or ½ stick) butter

½ lb. mushrooms, sliced

1 medium yellow onion, finely chopped

1 cup chopped tart green apple, peeled

2 lb. small (50- to 60-count) fresh shrimp, headed and cleaned

½ lb. lobster tail meat, cut into bite-size chunks

½ lb. lump white crabmeat

2 tsp. salt

Dash of freshly ground black pepper

1 slice (¼ in. thick) ginger root, minced

2 tsp. granulated sugar

3 cups chicken broth

2 cups coconut milk

3 TB. cornstarch stirred into 6 TB. water

2 TB. lemon juice

Paprika

Hot cooked rice

1. Melt 2 tablespoons butter in a large skillet over medium heat and sauté mushrooms and yellow onion until onion is translucent.

2. Add green apple and continue sautéing until apple is tender but not broken down. Spoon contents into a medium bowl and set aside.

3. Add remaining 2 tablespoons butter to the skillet along with shrimp, lobster tail meat, and lump white crabmeat. Sauté for 5 minutes or until shrimp are pink and lobster has developed its red coloring.

4. Return mushroom mixture to the skillet and add salt, black pepper, ginger root, and sugar. Stir to combine.

5. Stir in chicken broth and coconut milk and bring to a simmer.

6. Add cornstarch slurry and cook, stirring gently, until sauce thickens.

7. Remove from heat and stir in lemon juice.

8. Garnish with a sprinkle of paprika and serve hot over freshly prepared rice.

TROPICAL TIP

Frozen or canned seafood may be used, but fresh is definitely best!

Waikiki Coconut Shrimp

The hoisin sauce in this recipe lends an almond flavor to this dish. Oyster sauce can be substituted with equally good results in a different flavor profile.

Yield:	Prep time:	Cook time:	Serving size:
2 pounds	24 hours (marinate time)	60 minutes	½ pound

Each serving has:			
66.4 g carbohydrate	18.5 g fat	5.7 g fiber	45.5 g protein
12 g coconut oil = .8 TB.			

1½ lb. fresh large (25- to 30-count) or jumbo (20- to 25-count) shrimp, butterflied (leave tail fins on)	1 TB. sherry
	2 cups all-purpose flour
	¼ cup cornstarch
2 TB. plus 1 tsp. hoisin sauce	2 tsp. baking powder
1 TB. soy sauce	1 tsp. salt
1 slice (¼ in. thick) ginger root, minced	1 large egg, beaten
	1½ cups water
2 tsp. sesame oil	2 cups flaked coconut

1. Place shrimp in a shallow bowl and combine with 2 tablespoons hoisin sauce, soy sauce, ginger root, 1 teaspoon sesame oil, and sherry. Stir to coat shrimp well and allow to marinate overnight.

2. Combine all-purpose flour, cornstarch, baking powder, and salt in a medium bowl.

3. Combine remaining 1 teaspoon sesame oil, egg, water, and remaining 1 teaspoon hoisin sauce in a bowl and gradually add to flour mixture, stirring until batter is smooth and free of lumps.

4. One at a time and holding shrimp by the tail fins, remove shrimp from marinade and dip them into batter, and then roll in flaked coconut. Gently press coconut onto shrimp if necessary.

5. Place each shrimp on a greased baking sheet and refrigerate for 30 minutes to let batter set on shrimp.

6. In a large skillet, heat 1 inch of RBD or expeller-pressed coconut oil. Holding shrimp by the tail, place each in the skillet one at a time. Do not crowd the skillet.

7. Lower heat to medium and fry (in batches if necessary) until golden brown.

8. Place on a wire rack set on a baking sheet, in a warm oven set on lowest heat, until all have been fried.

TROPICAL TIP

Tempura shrimp can be prepared in advance by following the Waikiki Coconut Shrimp recipe and frying the shrimp only until they are lightly browned. Finish later by heating, covered, in a preheated 325°F oven for 10 minutes. Uncover to crisp and brown.

Aloha Lobster

This fresh island curry with spices echoes the flavors and aromas of Southeast Asia.

Yield:	Prep time:	Cook time:	Serving size:
6 cups	10 minutes	30 minutes	1 cup

Each serving has:			
9.6 g carbohydrate	18.6 g fat	1.9 g fiber	18 g protein
2.8 g coconut oil = .19 TB.			

4 TB. butter

2 medium onions, chopped

1 clove garlic, crushed and minced

2 tsp. curry powder

1 tsp. turmeric

2½ cups chicken broth

1 cup canned coconut milk

1 sliced (¼ in. thick) ginger

root, minced

1 tsp. salt

1 tsp. lemon juice

1 lb. lobster tail meat, cut into bite-size pieces

2 TB. cornstarch mixed into ¼ cup water

Hot cooked rice

1. Melt butter in a large skillet over medium heat and sauté onions and garlic until they have softened.

2. Add curry powder and turmeric and continue cooking and stirring for 1 minute more.

3. Stir in chicken broth, coconut milk, and ginger root and bring to a simmer.

4. Stir in salt, lemon juice, and lobster tail meat. Continue simmering for 10 minutes more.

5. When sauce is very hot, stir in cornstarch slurry and cook, continuing to stir until sauce thickens.

6. Serve over hot, freshly cooked rice.

Variation: Replace lobster meat with 2 pounds of headed and deveined medium (40– to 50-count) shrimp.

TO YOUR HEALTH!

To increase the coconut oil content of curries, serve them in bowls made of halved coconut shells. Find a friend to help you and simply saw young coconuts into halves using a handsaw. The pointed end will have to be trimmed as well so that the coconut bowl will sit upright.

Lanai Chicken Salad

This fresh-tasting, light salad makes a cool summer lunch for dining outside on your *lanai*, or it makes a nice side salad for a heavier evening meal.

Yield:	Prep time:	Serving size:
6 cups	5 minutes	1 cup

Each serving has:			
23.8 g carbohydrate	16.1 g fat	1.7 g fiber	28.2 g protein
40 g coconut oil = 2.66 TB.			

4 cups cooked chicken, diced

1½ cups celery, finely diced

½ small onion, grated

2 cups fresh green seedless grapes, halved

1 (13-oz.) can pineapple tidbits, drained well

1 cup plain coconut mayonnaise (see Herbed Mayonnaise recipe in Chapter 16)

Salt and freshly ground black pepper to taste

3 small coconuts, halved

1. In a medium mixing bowl, thoroughly combine chicken, celery, onion, green seedless grapes, pineapple, and coconut mayonnaise. Cover and chill for 30 minutes.

2. Taste for seasoning and adjust by adding salt and black pepper if desired.

3. Using a large spoon, heap salad into coconut shell halves. Serve cold.

DEFINITION

Lanai is the name of the sixth-largest island of the Hawaiian island chain. A **lanai** (lowercase) is an architectural feature of a home, consisting of a furnished outdoor patio that functions as a room. Lanais sometimes are completely open but may have roofs and often have removable screens or storm doors.

Sweet Potato Mock Poi

This mock *poi* recipe replaces taro root with sweet potatoes to please and appease the mainland palate.

Yield:	Prep time:	Cook time:	Serving size:
8 cups	5 minutes	15 minutes	¾ cup

Each serving has:			
44 g carbohydrate	9.8 g fat	7 g fiber	3.2 g protein
2.8 g coconut oil = .19 TB.			

6 large sweet potatoes, peeled, cubed, and boiled until tender

¼ tsp. salt

¼ tsp. freshly ground black pepper

1 cup canned coconut milk

1. In a large mixing bowl, mash together sweet potatoes with salt and black pepper.

2. Gradually beat in coconut milk until mixture results in the desired consistency.

3. Serve as a side dish in individual bowls.

DEFINITION

Poi is a traditional, tangy, fermented Hawaiian food made of taro root, and many mainlanders never develop a taste for it. The consistency of the poi is indicated by its name—one-finger poi can be scooped up and eaten using one finger, two-finger poi is thinner and requires two fingers, and so on.

Samoan-Style Baked Spinach

Have your own luau with this Samoan-style side dish, which replaces difficult-to-find taro leaves with the warm, familiar flavor of freshly cooked spinach.

Yield:	Prep time:	Cook time:	Serving size:
6 cups	10 minutes	30 minutes	1 cup

Each serving has:			
9.9 g carbohydrate	19.7 g fat	5.1 g fiber	6.2 g protein
19.1 g coconut oil = 1.3 TB.			

2 lb. fresh spinach	2 cups coconut cream
1 tsp. salt	

1. Rinse and dry spinach. Remove any tough stems.

2. Place spinach in a baking dish along with salt and coconut cream. Stir to combine.

3. Bake at 300°F about 30 minutes or until spinach is tender.

TO YOUR HEALTH!

Luau means "cooked taro leaf." Okay, for some people it also means "party," but the traditional Hawaiian luau is named for the cooked leaf of the taro plant. Taro leaves (also known as elephant ears) are rich in vitamins and minerals, but it is important to know that *raw* taro leaves are toxic. Popular in Pacific Island cuisines, these leaves are often eaten steamed or as a wrap for other foods.

Island-Style Coconut Rice

Coconut rice goes well with any spicy or fragrant curry.

Yield:	Prep time:	Cook time:	Serving size:
4 cups	5 minutes	30 minutes	⅔ cup

Each serving has:			
56.5 g carbohydrate	33.2 g fat	3.5 g fiber	7.2 g protein
11 g coconut oil = .73 TB.			

1 TB. butter	2 cups uncooked rice
½ small yellow onion, chopped	3 cups coconut milk
1 TB. coconut oil	

1. Melt butter in a medium saucepan over medium heat. Add yellow onion and sauté until golden. Remove onions and reserve.

2. Add coconut oil and rice to the saucepan and sauté for 1 to 2 minutes until rice takes on a whiter appearance.

3. Pour in coconut milk and bring to a simmer.

4. Cover the saucepan and reduce heat to medium-low. Allow rice to cook, covered, for 20 minutes.

5. When rice is done, stir in reserved onions and serve hot.

AW, NUTS!

Brown rice is healthier than polished white rice because it retains much of its vitamin-rich bran and germ, while white rice is left with only the starchy endosperm. When substituting brown rice for white, be sure to allow sufficient cooking time. Whereas white rice will finish cooking in 18 to 20 minutes, brown rice needs to cook for 45 minutes or more.

Fried Brown Rice (Traditional Indian Cuisine)

Indian-style fried brown rice is a delicately sweet and highly aromatic accompaniment to any richly flavored main course.

Yield:	Prep time:	Cook time:	Serving size:
3 cups	30 minutes (soaking time)	25 minutes	½ cup

Each serving has:			
33.8 g carbohydrate	10 g fat	.5 g fiber	2.8 g protein
10 g coconut oil = .67 TB.			

1¼ cups uncooked long-grain white rice, such as basmati	6 whole cloves
¼ cup coconut oil	6 black peppercorns
4 tsp. granulated sugar	2 bay leaves
1 tsp. cumin seeds	2½ cups water
2 (2-in.) cinnamon sticks, broken into small pieces	1 tsp. salt

1. Rinse long-grain white rice, cover with cold water, and allow soak to for 30 minutes. Drain well.

2. In a medium heavy-bottomed saucepan or Dutch oven, heat coconut oil over medium heat and add sugar.

3. Sugar will begin to change color, going from white to dark brown. As soon this happens, add cumin seeds, cinnamon pieces, cloves, black peppercorns, and bay leaves. Cook, stirring constantly, for 30 seconds.

4. Add rice and continue to cook and stir-fry about 5 minutes more. Lower heat during the last couple of minutes so that the rice and spices do not burn.

5. Add water and salt.

6. Bring to a boil and cover.

7. Reduce heat to a simmer and cook without lifting the lid (12 to 15 minutes for basmati rice, 18 to 20 minutes for other long-grain rice, or adjust cooking time according to your rice package's cooking instructions).

8. Do not remove the lid, but set the pan aside to rest for a further 10 to 15 minutes.

9. Remove bay leaves and any larger pieces of cinnamon sticks before serving. Serve immediately.

> **TO YOUR HEALTH!**
>
> In addition to healthy coconut oil, the cuisines of the tropics use lots of healthy aromatic herbs and spices, most of which have very high levels of antioxidants and healing properties of their own. Among them are ginger root, turmeric, cilantro, onion, garlic, hot chile peppers, citrus fruits and juices, pineapple, mango, and papaya.

Indian-Style Coconut Pancakes (Dosas)

Dosas are crispy, savory *idli* pancakes from Southern India that can be eaten alone or used as a base or wrap for any number of foods.

Yield:	Prep time:	Cook time:	Serving size:
20 pancakes	2 days	30 minutes	2 pancakes

Each serving has:			
45.6 g carbohydrate	6.6 g fat	9.1 g fiber	8.7 g protein
4.8 g coconut oil = .32 TB.			

1 cup lentils	2 small green chiles, coarsely chopped
2 TB. lemon juice	2 small onions, coarsely chopped
Warm water	
2 cups brown rice	1 bunch cilantro
1½ tsp. salt	⅓ cup coconut oil
2 cups finely grated coconut	
2 TB. fresh ginger root, coarsely chopped	

1. Rinse lentils well and place in a bowl. Stir in 1 tablespoon lemon juice, add warm water just to cover, and set aside.

2. Place brown rice in a separate bowl, add remaining 1 tablespoon lemon juice and warm water just to cover, and set aside.

3. Allow lentils and rice to soak in a warm place overnight.

4. Drain lentils and purée in a food processor (adding a little water as necessary) until completely smooth.

5. Repeat with rice.

6. Combine puréed lentils and rice, along with 1 teaspoon salt and enough water to create a batter that resembles the thickness of cream.

7. Cover with a clean dish towel and set aside in a warm place for 24 hours more.

8. Place coconut, ginger root, green chiles, onions, cilantro, and remaining ½ teaspoon salt in a food processor.

9. Process until a paste forms.

10. Stir mixture into lentil and rice batter until well combined, adding additional water as necessary to create a creamy pancake batter.

11. Heat a heavy-bottomed medium skillet and brush it generously with coconut oil.

12. Ladle ¼ cup batter onto the hot skillet and swirl the pan slightly to help the batter spread.

13. Cook 5 minutes per side or until pancake has fully cooked through, brushing more coconut oil on skillet surface between each pancake.

14. Serve warm with curry, fruit chutney, hummus, or a tangy yogurt sauce.

DEFINITION

Idli foods are acidified and leavened by lactic acid bacteria in much the same way sourdough bread is produced but without the need for wheat or rye proteins. Because of its acidity, the idli fermentation process protects against food poisoning and the transfer of pathogenic organisms. And because they are easily digested, they are often use as food for babies or the infirm.

Baba Ghanoush

This Middle Eastern appetizer or side dish boasts a wonderful balance of flavor and texture defined by creamy, smoky eggplant contrasted with bright lemon and garlic. Tahini lends it some body, while the coconut oil makes for an exotic finish.

Yield:	Prep time:	Cook time:	Serving size:
2 cups	5 minutes	45 minutes	2 tablespoons

Each serving has:			
7 g carbohydrate	8 g fat	1 g fiber	15.2 g protein
4.33 g coconut oil = .29 TB.			

1 large eggplant	2 garlic cloves, crushed and peeled
¼ cup virgin coconut oil	¼ cup tahini
Salt	Extra-virgin olive oil (optional)
Coarsely ground black pepper	
3 TB. fresh lemon juice	

1. Cut eggplant in half lengthwise. Without piercing the skin, score-cut surface of each half ½-inch deep in a diamond pattern from edge to edge.

2. Brush each scored surface with 1 tablespoon virgin coconut oil.

3. Sprinkle liberally with salt and black pepper and place cut side down on a cookie sheet.

4. Roast in a 350°F oven for 45 minutes or until flesh is very soft. Set aside and allow eggplant to cool before handling.

5. With a large spoon, scoop out flesh and purée in a food processor along with lemon juice, garlic, and tahini until smooth.

6. Add remaining virgin coconut oil and blend in. Taste for salt and pepper, adjusting seasoning if necessary.

7. Serve in a large dip bowl alongside a variety of crudités and pita chips.

8. Drizzle with extra-virgin olive oil (if using).

TROPICAL TIP

Baba ganoush is typically served with warm pita bread and an assortment of crudités.

Soups, Curries, and Condiments

In This Chapter

- Healthy, easy "go-to" meals
- Make mealtimes exotic
- Expand your possibilities using classic base sauces and condiments
- Last-minute tips

Soups are as old as the history of cooking itself. That's because there is nothing easier or more nourishing than a homemade soup made with fresh ingredients. In fact, every traditional culture on earth has known this and has developed distinctive soups from fresh ingredients suited to the growing conditions of its particular climate.

Native tropical foods like the coconut, plus its milk, oil, and cream, make some of the very healthiest soups ever created, and they come together to produce the taste sensations and exotic aromas we associate with traditional Thai, Indian, and island cuisines.

As promised, this chapter will introduce you to some coconut soup and curry favorites, but we won't stop there. After experimenting with a few basic recipes for creamy velouté, aioli, and herbed mayonnaise, you'll soon be creating brand new coconut dishes to showcase your own unique style and cooking flair.

Before You Put the Soup On …

Since coconut is most widely used in the cuisines of Asia and the South Pacific, you may be unfamiliar with some of the ingredients and terms in this chapter. But rest assured, sources for ingredients are included in Appendix B, and any unusual terms are defined within the recipes and listed again in Appendix A for easy reference.

If you aren't able to find a particular ingredient, please don't let that stop you from having some fun. I encourage you to either omit the ingredient altogether or try substituting something similar. These recipes are very forgiving!

Chilled Coconut Soup

This refreshing, chilled soup works well served after a spicy appetizer course by deliciously cooling and cleansing the palate.

Yield:	Prep time:	Cook time:	Serving size:
10 cups	45 minutes (including chill time)	40 minutes	1½ cups

Each serving has:			
20.2 g carbohydrate 39.3 g fat 1.88 g coconut oil = .72 TB.		4.7 g fiber	10 g protein

5 cups milk	½ tsp. salt
2⅔ cups dried unsweetened shredded coconut	½ tsp. freshly ground black pepper
1⅔ cups coconut milk	1 tsp. granulated sugar
1⅔ cups chicken stock	1 small bunch fresh cilantro, finely chopped
1 cup heavy cream	

1. Pour milk into a large heavy-bottomed saucepan.

2. Stirring constantly over medium-high heat, bring milk to a moderate boil.

3. Stir in unsweetened coconut, lower heat, and allow soup to simmer for about 30 minutes.

4. Remove from heat and, using a submersion blender or food processor, blend soup until it is very smooth, pausing to scrape down the sides of the pan or bowl as necessary.

5. Return soup to the burner and stir in coconut milk, chicken stock, heavy cream, salt, black pepper, and sugar.

6. While stirring, bring soup back to a boil, then lower heat and simmer for about 10 minutes more.

7. Add chopped cilantro to taste.

8. Remove soup to a large bowl and allow it to cool.

9. Cover soup and place in the refrigerator to chill.

10. When fully chilled, taste and adjust seasoning if necessary.

11. Serve garnished with a few fresh cilantro leaves in pre-chilled bowls.

TROPICAL TIP

Chilled coconut soup is the perfect choice for a light meal on a hot summer day.

Spicy Thai Soup with Coconut Milk

The flavor profile of this soup is both balanced and complex, with the cooling qualities of cucumber, mint, and coconut milk providing the perfect counterpoint to the jalapeño's heat.

Yield:	Prep time:	Cook time:	Serving size:
8 cups	10 minutes	40 minutes	2 cups

Each serving has:			
168.4 g carbohydrate 25.4 g fat		6.7 g fiber	22.9 g protein
11.2 g coconut oil = .75 TB.			

½ cup cucumber, diced

1 jalapeño pepper, halved, seeded, and finely sliced

½ cup fresh mint, roughly chopped

1 cup fresh mung bean sprouts, rinsed and drained

½ cup fresh cilantro leaves, roughly chopped

½ lb. firm tofu, cubed

4 cups cooked medium-grain rice

1 small yellow or red onion, chopped

5 cloves garlic, minced

2 stalks lemongrass, trimmed to 1-in. pieces

2-in. knob fresh ginger root, peeled and sliced

2 or 3 fresh red chile peppers, chopped

1 tsp. ground cumin

1 TB. ground coriander

½ tsp. turmeric

2 tsp. brown rice syrup

2 TB. coconut oil

5 cups water

¼ cup fresh lime juice

1 (14-oz.) can coconut milk

1 tsp. sea salt

1 fresh lime, quartered (optional)

1. Lightly mix cucumber, jalapeño pepper, mint, mung bean sprouts, cilantro, and tofu together in a medium bowl and set aside.

2. Evenly divide cooked rice among 4 large soup bowls and set aside.

3. To make soup stock, place yellow onion, garlic, lemongrass, ginger root, red chile peppers, cumin, coriander, turmeric, and brown rice syrup in a food processor and process until it forms a paste.

4. Heat coconut oil in a heavy-bottomed Dutch oven, but don't allow it to smoke.

5. While stirring constantly, pour paste into hot oil and sauté for about 5 to 7 minutes.

6. Stir in water, lime juice, coconut milk, and sea salt and bring stock to a boil.

7. Lower the heat and allow soup stock to simmer for about 30 minutes longer.

8. While retaining liquid, strain soup stock using a kitchen sieve and discard solid ingredients.

9. Rinse the pot to remove any solids and return liquid soup base to it. Keep stock over low heat until soup is served.

10. To serve soup, ladle hot stock over each bowl of prepared rice.

11. Mound equal amounts of vegetable/tofu mixture in the center of each soup bowl.

12. Garnish by topping each bowl with a fresh lime wedge (if using) and serve immediately.

TROPICAL TIP

This exotic soup is simple to prepare and takes less than an hour to put together. Most of your energy will be spent in basic prep, though, so assemble your ingredients first and then get started!

Vegetarian Butternut Squash Soup

Dreamy, creamy butternut squash soup is actually a very mild coconut milk curry. Let the intoxicating flavors and aromas of warm coconut, ginger, turmeric, cumin, and cilantro transport you to the Middle East for dinner tonight!

Yield:	Prep time:	Cook time:	Serving size:
12 cups	10 minutes	30 minutes	1½ cups

Each serving has:			
18.9 g carbohydrate	16.6 g fat	3.8 g fiber	6.4 g protein
5.67 g coconut oil = .37 TB.			

2 TB. coconut oil	2 tsp. ground cumin
1 large yellow onion, chopped	1 medium butternut squash, peeled, seeded, and cut into ½-in. cubes
1-in. knob fresh ginger root, peeled and minced	
6 cloves garlic, crushed and minced	1 (14-oz.) can coconut milk
	Salt
6 cups organic chicken or vegetable broth	Freshly ground black pepper
2 tsp. turmeric	¼ cup fresh cilantro, chopped

1. In a medium stockpot, melt coconut oil and sauté yellow onion over medium heat until translucent. Do not allow onion to brown.

2. Add ginger root and garlic to onion and continue sautéing mixture for another minute or so.

3. Add chicken broth, turmeric, cumin, and butternut squash to the stockpot, stirring to combine.

4. Raise heat to high and bring soup to a boil. Reduce heat to low and continue to cook uncovered for about 10 minutes or until the squash is tender.

5. Stir coconut milk into soup.

6. Using a blender, food processor, or submersion (stick) blender, purée soup until it is completely smooth.

7. Season to taste with salt and black pepper.

8. Stir in cilantro and reheat soup if necessary. Serve hot.

Variation: Cool soup in the refrigerator and then blend in the flesh of 1 ripe avocado. Serve chilled.

TROPICAL TIP

When cleaning winter squash, save the seeds and toast them in the oven to make a healthy snack or garnish for soups and salads. Squash seeds are an excellent, heart-healthy snack full of magnesium and fiber.

Thai-Style Lentil and Coconut Soup

This filling soup boasts all the heat, spice, rich flavors, and aroma that have made healthy Thai cuisine famous.

Yield:	Prep time:	Cook time:	Serving size:
6 cups	10 minutes	1 hour	1½ cups

Each serving has:			
42 g carbohydrate	18.5 g fiber	31.2 g fat	15.8 g protein
11.22 g coconut oil = .75 TB.			

2 TB. coconut oil	1 tsp. paprika
2 medium red onions, finely chopped	1 (14-oz.) can coconut milk
1 Thai chile, seeded and finely sliced	3¾ cups water
	Juice of 1 lime
2 cloves garlic, crushed and minced	3 whole green onions, sliced (reserve some for garnish)
1-in. piece fresh lemongrass (inner layers only), finely sliced	½ bunch fresh cilantro, finely chopped (reserve some for garnish)
1 cup uncooked split red lentils	Salt
1 tsp. ground coriander	Freshly ground black pepper

1. Melt coconut oil in a medium stockpot and add red onions, Thai chile, garlic, and lemongrass.

2. Sauté over medium heat until onions have softened.

3. Add red lentils, coriander, paprika, coconut milk, and water.

4. While stirring, bring soup to a boil.

5. Reduce the heat and allow to simmer for about 45 minutes or until lentils have softened and are fully cooked.

6. Remove soup from heat.

7. Finish by stirring in lime juice, green onions, and cilantro.

8. Adjust seasoning with salt and black pepper to taste.

9. Serve hot, garnished with a little freshly sliced green onion and fresh cilantro leaves.

TROPICAL TIP

Offer diners a basket of warm naan or pita bread to make this hearty soup into a complete meal. Naan is a round leavened flatbread that accompanies most meals in many regions of South and Central Asia—especially India. It is also commonly eaten in Afghanistan, Iran, Pakistan, and Uzbekistan.

Indian-Style Lamb Soup with Coconut and Rice

This soup is based on mulligatawny (literally, "pepper water") soup, a true classic in Indian cuisine. This version is enhanced by the warm flavors and aromas of cumin and coriander and is thickened with rice.

Yield:	Prep time:	Cook time:	Serving size:
8 cups	15 minutes	1 hour	1½ cups

Each serving has:			
14.8 g carbohydrate	23.1 g fat	1.5 g fiber	25.2 g protein
15.7 g coconut oil = 1.05 TB.			

2 medium yellow onions, chopped	5 cups lamb or beef stock
6 cloves garlic, crushed	¼ tsp. cayenne
2-in. knob fresh ginger root, very finely minced or grated	⅓ cup uncooked long-grain white rice, such as basmati
6 TB. coconut oil	¼ cup coconut milk
2 TB. black poppy seeds	2 TB. lemon juice
1 tsp. cumin seeds	Salt
1 tsp. coriander seeds	Coarsely ground black pepper
½ tsp. ground turmeric	6 fresh cilantro sprigs
1 lb. lamb stew meat, trimmed and cut to bite-size chunks	Flaked unsweetened coconut, toasted

1. Using a food processor or blender, process yellow onions, garlic, and ginger root together with 1 tablespoon coconut oil. Set this paste aside.

2. In a medium heavy-bottomed pot or Dutch oven, toast black poppy seeds, cumin seeds, and coriander seeds until they begin to become fragrant. Then grind toasted seeds using a mortar and pestle or in an electric coffee or spice mill.

3. Stir turmeric into ground seeds and set spices aside.

4. Brown lamb stew meat using the same heavy-bottomed pan and remaining 5 tablespoons coconut oil, in batches if necessary, for about 5 minutes. Remove meat and set aside.

5. Put onions, garlic, and ginger paste into the pan and cook, stirring constantly, for a minute or two. Then add ground spices and continue cooking for about 1 minute more.

6. Return meat and its juices to the pan, along with lamb stock and cayenne. Bring liquid to a boil, reduce the heat, cover, and simmer until lamb is tender—about 30 minutes.

7. Stir in the uncooked long-grain rice, cover, and continue to cook at a medium simmer for another 20 minutes or until rice is tender.

8. Stir in coconut milk and lemon juice. Taste for salt and black pepper, adjusting if necessary, and cook a little longer so that whole soup is warmed through.

9. Serve soup piping hot, garnished with a fresh sprig of cilantro and toasted coconut flakes.

TROPICAL TIP

Although there are quite a few steps involved in the preparation of this dish, having all your ingredients assembled and measured before you begin makes this soup come together like a breeze!

Coconut and Seafood Soup

Green curry paste, ginger, lemongrass, and kaffir lime lend an interesting complexity to the rich seafood undertones of this dish.

Yield:	Prep time:	Cook time:	Serving size:
6 cups	25 minutes	30 minutes	1½ cups

Each serving has:			
102 g carbohydrate	32.1 g fat	2.7 g fiber	47.7 g protein
7.47 g coconut oil = .5 TB.			

5 or 6 (¼ in. thick) slices fresh ginger root

2 lemongrass stalks, chopped

3 kaffir lime leaves, *chiffonade*

1 bunch garlic chives

2½ cups fish stock

½ bunch fresh cilantro

1 TB. coconut oil

4 shallots, chopped

3 TB. Thai fish sauce

1 lb. fresh medium (40– to 50-count) shrimp, headed, peeled, and deveined

4 TB. Thai green curry paste

1 lb. prepared fresh squid

Fresh lime juice

Salt

Coarsely ground black pepper

¼ cup canned French fried onions

1. Place the ginger root, lemongrass, half of kaffir lime leaves, and half of garlic chives in a stockpot along with fish stock. Reserve remaining kaffir lime leaves and garlic chives for later.

2. Separate cilantro leaves from their stalks and place stalks in stock, reserving leaves for later.

3. Bring stock to a boil, cover, and reduce the heat to low, allowing the pot to simmer for 30 minutes.

4. Using a colander or kitchen sieve, strain stock into a large bowl.

5. Wipe the stockpot dry. Add coconut oil and chopped shallots to the pot and sauté until shallots are a golden color.

6. Add back strained stock along with remaining kaffir lime leaves and 2 table-spoons of Thai fish sauce.

7. Bring to a medium simmer and continue to cook over gentle heat for about 10 minutes more.

8. Stir in cleaned shrimp and Thai green curry paste and cook for 3 minutes.

9. Add squid and cook for 2 minutes more. Finish by adding lime juice.

10. Taste for seasoning and add salt and black pepper if necessary.

11. Taste for seasoning, adding additional fish sauce if necessary. Stir in cilantro leaves and serve garnished with French fried onions and remaining garlic chives.

Variation: Substitute 14 ounces of firm white fish cut into bite-size pieces for the squid.

DEFINITION

Chiffonade is a technique for cutting leafy herbs into long fine ribbons. Simply stack the leaves, roll them tightly, and cut thin slices from the roll to produce the thin strips of herbs.

Thai-Style Pumpkin, Shrimp, and Coconut Soup

The natural sweetness of pumpkin is balanced by chiles, shrimp, and coconut cream in this beautiful soup.

Yield:	Prep time:	Cook time:	Serving size:
10 cups	30 minutes	1 hour	$1\frac{1}{2}$ cups

Each serving has:			
13.2 g carbohydrate	24.5 g fat	4.4 g fiber	7.7 g protein
23.8 g coconut oil = 1.6 TB.			

2 cloves garlic, crushed and minced	$2\frac{1}{2}$ cups coconut cream
4 shallots, finely chopped	2 TB. Thai fish sauce
$\frac{1}{2}$ tsp. shrimp paste	1 tsp. granulated sugar
1 lemongrass stalk, chopped	$\frac{1}{4}$ tsp. salt
2 fresh green chiles, seeded	$\frac{1}{4}$ tsp. freshly ground black pepper
1 TB. dried shrimp, soaked in warm water	4 oz. small (50- to 60-count) salad shrimp, precooked
$2\frac{1}{2}$ cups chicken stock	2 fresh red chiles, seeded and finely sliced
1 lb. pumpkin, peeled, seeded, and cubed	Fresh basil leaves

1. Place garlic, shallots, shrimp paste, lemongrass, and green chiles in a food processor.

2. Discarding water, drain soaked shrimp and add to the food processor. Process ingredients until a paste forms.

3. Pour chicken stock into a Dutch oven, add processed paste, and bring stock to a boil over medium-high heat. Stir until paste is dissolved.

4. Add pumpkin chunks and simmer 15 minutes or until pumpkin is fork-tender.

5. Stir in coconut cream, Thai fish sauce, sugar, salt, and black pepper while continuing to simmer a few minutes more.

6. Add salad shrimp and simmer 1 minute more or until shrimp are heated through.

7. Serve hot, garnished with red chiles and fresh basil leaves.

TO YOUR HEALTH!

Shrimp paste is a traditional lacto-fermented food made by allowing shrimp to ferment in a salty brine. Lacto-fermentation is achieved by live *lactobacillus* bacteria that add to the healthy flora in our gut.

Chicken, Ginger, and Coconut Soup

Ginger root, lemongrass, and kaffir lime wake up the palate and stimulate the senses.

Yield:	Prep time:	Cook time:	Serving size:
10 cup	30 minutes	45 minutes	1½ cups

Each serving has:			
9.5 g carbohydrate	29.7 g fat	3.2 g fiber	17.3 g protein
13.5 g coconut oil = .9 TB.			

3 cups coconut milk

2 cups chicken stock

4 lemongrass stalks, bruised and chopped

1-in. piece ginger root, peeled and julienne sliced

10 black peppercorns

10 kaffir lime leaves, roughly torn

¾ lb. boneless, skinless chicken breast strips

4 oz. fresh white mushrooms (about 1 cup sliced, or about 15 whole)

½ cup baby corncobs

4 TB. lime juice

3 TB. Thai fish sauce

2 red Thai chiles, chopped

4 green onions, sliced

½ cup fresh cilantro, roughly chopped

1. Pour coconut milk and chicken stock into a medium stockpot and bring to a boil over medium-high heat.

2. Add lemongrass, ginger root, black peppercorns, and half of kaffir lime leaves. Reduce heat and simmer 10 minutes.

3. Strain stock into a clean Dutch oven and add chicken strips, mushrooms, and corncobs. Cook over medium heat 10 minutes or until chicken is cooked through and tender.

4. Stir in lime juice, Thai fish sauce, and remaining kaffir lime leaves.

5. Serve immediately, garnished with a sprinkle of red chiles, green onions, and cilantro.

TROPICAL TIP

Always take care when working with fresh chiles. Their volatile oils can burn the skin and eyes. Their heat and flavor will transfer from the surfaces of knives and cutting boards to other foods, too.

Brazilian Crab, Coconut, and Cilantro Soup (Moqueca)

Creamy coconut, palm oil, fragrant cilantro, and chiles define the flavor profile of this Brazilian warmer.

Yield:	Prep time:	Cook time:	Serving size:
8 cups	10 minutes	30 minutes	1⅓ cups

Each serving has:			
20.8 g carbohydrate	16 g fat	1.9 g fiber	25.8 g protein
2.8 g coconut oil = .19 TB.			

2 TB. olive oil	4 cups crab or fish stock
1 medium yellow onion, finely chopped	1½ lb. crabmeat (lump, white is best)
1 rib celery, finely chopped	1 cup coconut milk
2 cloves garlic, crushed	2 TB. red palm oil
1 fresh red chile, seeded and chopped	Juice of 1 fresh lime
	½ tsp. salt
1 large tomato, chopped	Hot chile oil
¼ cup fresh cilantro, chopped	Lime wedges

1. Pour olive oil into a medium stockpot and sauté onion and celery over medium-low heat for 5 minutes or until onion is translucent.

2. Add garlic and red chile and sauté for 2 minutes more.

3. Add tomato and half of cilantro, stirring to warm tomato through.

4. Pour in crab stock and bring to a boil. Lower heat and simmer for 5 minutes.

5. Stir in crabmeat, coconut milk, and red palm oil. Continue to simmer for 5 minutes more.

6. Remove from heat. Stir in lime juice and salt.

7. Serve moqueca garnished with several drops of hot chile oil, a lime wedge, and remaining cilantro as desired.

DEFINITION

Moqueca, in the Afro-Brazilian cuisine of Bahia, is a regional specialty soup. Usually made with fresh coconut milk, shrimp, malagueta peppers, and dendê oil. Traditionally, it is cooked very slowly over low heat to retain all the vital nutrients of the food.

Velouté Base for a Nondairy Cream Soup

This velouté is a velvety smooth sauce that takes on and echoes the flavors of the foods cooked with it.

Yield:	Prep time:	Cook time:	Serving size:
4 cups	2 minutes	10 minutes	²/₃ cup
Each serving has:			
8.7 g carbohydrate	145.33 g fat	4 g fiber	5.3 g protein
48 g coconut oil = 3.2 TB.			

4 cups chicken stock	¹/₂ tsp. sea salt
2 cups coconut cream concentrate (also known as coconut butter)	¹/₄ tsp. black pepper, fresh and coarsely ground

1. Combine chicken stock and coconut cream concentrate in a large saucepan.

2. Increase heat and continue stirring until mixture comes to a boil.

3. Stir in sea salt and black pepper. Reduce heat and allow to simmer 2 to 3 minutes.

4. Use as a base for creamy mushroom, vegetable, or seafood soups and sauces.

Variation: Use velouté as a soup base. While the velouté is simmering, stir in your soup's main ingredients. Continue cooking until the vegetables are tender and any seafood is just done. Taste and adjust seasoning as necessary. Serve hot.

> **TROPICAL TIP**
>
> A velouté is one of the five "mother sauces" in classical French cuisine. It serves as a versatile base for many soups and other sauces. In this recipe, coconut cream concentrate substitutes for the traditional butter and flour roux.
>
> Veloutés work well with many combinations of ingredients. Try pairing your favorite vegetable medley with fresh seafood or prepared veal or chicken. Your imagination is the limit, so try all your favorites.

Aioli

Serve distinctive, garlicky aioli anytime to add zest to otherwise ordinary foods.

Yield:	Prep time:	Serving size:	
2 cups	7 minutes	1 tablespoon	
Each serving has:			
1.2 g carbohydrate	11.1 g fat	0 g fiber	.7 g protein
11 g coconut oil = .74 TB.			

1 chunk stale French bread (enough to yield ⅓ cup dry breadcrumbs)

2 TB. white wine vinegar

6 or 8 cloves garlic, crushed

½ tsp. salt

6 egg yolks

1 TB. fresh lemon juice

1 TB. fish stock or water

¼ tsp. freshly ground black pepper

¼ tsp. hot sauce

1½ cups coconut oil

1. Using a blender or food processor, prepare and measure French breadcrumbs.

2. Place measured breadcrumbs back into the blender along with white wine vinegar, garlic, salt, egg yolks, lemon juice, fish stock, black pepper, and hot sauce.

3. With the motor running, very slowly drizzle in coconut oil to create an emulsion. When done, aioli should resemble the consistency of mayonnaise.

> **TROPICAL TIP**
>
> If the aioli is too thick for your liking, blend in additional water or fish stock 1 tablespoon at a time until the correct consistency is achieved. Refrigerate leftovers in a tightly covered container and use within a couple of days.

Herbed Mayonnaise

Dress up your favorite sandwich or veggie dish with the flavors of your favorite herbs in this fresh-tasting mayonnaise.

Yield:	Prep time:	Cook time:	Serving size:
1 cup	7 minutes	1 minute	1 tablespoon

Each serving has:			
.3 g carbohydrate	13.9 g fat	0 g fiber	.4 g protein
13 g coconut oil = .9 TB.			

Fresh herbs of your choice (such as basil, parsley, cilantro, or chives—or a combination, such as the Italian herbs or herbes de Provence)

1 egg

½ tsp. salt

½ tsp. dry mustard

½ tsp. granulated sugar

Dash cayenne

2 TB. white wine vinegar, tarragon vinegar, or fresh lemon juice

1 cup coconut oil

1. Take a couple handfuls of fresh herbs and blanch them for 1 minute in boiling water.

2. Quickly remove herbs to an ice-water bath.

3. When chilled, remove herbs, dry, and mince finely. Set aside.

4. Place egg, salt, dry mustard, sugar, cayenne, and white wine vinegar in the blender.

5. Cover and begin processing.

6. Open the feeder cap and slowly drizzle in coconut oil at a steady rate to create an emulsion. (If necessary, stop the blender and use a rubber spatula to keep mixture around the blades. Then cover and continue to process until all of oil has been fully incorporated.)

7. Add minced herbs to the blender and pulse-blend until thoroughly combined.

8. Store covered in the refrigerator for up to 1 week.

Variation: For plain mayonnaise, simply leave out the herbs.

TO YOUR HEALTH!

Culinary herbs have been utilized throughout history in many interesting and beneficial ways to promote wellness, and their role in promoting good digestion is chief among them. Use herbs liberally to enhance food flavors and enjoy improved health, too.

Basic Vinaigrette

Vinaigrettes are versatile dressings that brighten the flavors of fresh salad ingredients.

Yield:	Prep time:	Serving size:
1 cup	5 minutes	1 tablespoon

Each serving has:			
0 g carbohydrate	10 g fat	0 g fiber	0 g protein
5.6 g coconut oil = .38 TB.			

¼ cup red wine vinegar	6 TB. coconut oil
Pinch salt	6 TB. extra-virgin olive oil
¼ tsp. freshly ground black pepper	

1. In a small mixing bowl, whisk together red wine vinegar, salt, and black pepper until salt is completely dissolved.

2. If coconut oil is solid, gently warm it until it melts. Combine coconut oil and extra-virgin olive oil in a measuring cup.

3. While continuously whisking vinegar, slowly drizzle in oils in a fine, steady stream until all of oil has been incorporated.

4. Always warm to room temperature and whisk again just before using.

Variation: To make **Garlic Vinaigrette,** add ½ teaspoon minced garlic in step 2. Allow garlic to rest in warm coconut oil for 30 minutes before proceeding.

For **Mustard Vinaigrette,** whisk 2 teaspoons Dijon mustard into the vinegar in step 1. Proceed with recipe as written.

For **Tarragon Vinaigrette**, stir 1 tablespoon fresh minced tarragon (or 2 teaspoons dried) into the finished Basic Vinaigrette recipe.

TO YOUR HEALTH!

Using homemade coconut oil–based salad dressings avoids the thyroid-damaging effects of soy-based commercial dressings and condiments.

Pineapple Coconut Sauce

Serve this tasty dipping sauce with tempura fried shrimp or chicken breast tenders.

Yield:	Prep time:	Cook time:	Serving size:
4 cups	5 minutes	5 minutes	⅔ cup

Each serving has:			
47.6 g carbohydrate	3.7 g fat	1.7 g fiber	1 g protein
2 g coconut oil = .13 TB.			

3 cups pineapple juice	Dash salt
½ cup granulated sugar	2 TB. honey
2 tsp. butter	½ cup flaked coconut
1 (13-oz.) can crushed pineapple	

1. In a medium saucepan, heat and stir together pineapple juice, sugar, and butter until sugar is completely dissolved.

2. Add crushed pineapple, salt, honey, and coconut.

3. Bring to a boil, reduce heat, and simmer for 5 minutes.

4. Serve hot.

TROPICAL TIP

Pineapple Coconut Sauce can be made ahead of time and stored, covered, in the refrigerator for several days. Simply reheat before serving. Keep some on hand for jazzing up a ho-hum meal, serving on ice cream, or glazing roasted meats.

Meals and Treats Especially for Dementia Patients

In This Chapter

- The importance of easy nutrition
- Providing good-quality meals for people with dementia
- Treats that are easy to digest

Caregivers of people who suffer from dementia learn soon enough that their loved ones are changing in unexpected ways. As time goes on, they develop special needs and, sometimes, astonishing new tastes as well.

While the recipes in this chapter are delightful meals and treats that anyone would enjoy, they have been especially selected with the needs of caregivers and dementia patients in mind. In the course of choosing which recipes to include, I have placed special emphasis on ease of preparation, healthful ingredients, and the dementia patient's sweet tooth and ability to handle or manipulate the food.

It's a sobering fact that, although we do everything in our power to slow and even reverse the progression of disorders like Alzheimer's disease, for now, dementias are still chronic and progressive in nature. Just like adjusting to the obvious mental changes, adjustments to the menu will be required.

The Quality and Qualities of Food

All foods give us four principal quality factors that many folks may not consciously consider:

- Appearance
- Texture
- Flavor and aroma
- Nutrition

Yet over time, an appealing appearance or packaging, whether a food is hard or soft, whether foods are finger foods or have sweet flavors, the quality of foods' nutrition, and the viscosity of liquids becomes more and more important to those with dementia. What works today may not work next week—and *will not* work in the *same way* next year.

The dementias are chronic progressive disease states—and they are still considered terminal. The patient changes drastically over time—sometimes in fits and starts, sometimes rapidly. There are good days, better days, difficult days, and *really* difficult days—and decline is inevitable. What your loved one craves and enjoys in the beginning of the dementia journey, he will find repugnant at a later date. What he can now manage to feed himself and chew and swallow without choking will change over time. Maybe his favorite fruit is strawberries, but now he has become afraid of the color red. Very often the demented become afraid of certain foods, or whoever is responsible for serving them, because they believe they are being poisoned. Every day (sometimes minute to minute), caregivers must learn new work-arounds.

A Bag of Tricks

Equally important is the caregiver's time. Caregiving is a 24/7 job with no vacation benefits and very few coffee breaks. Healthy recipes that come together quickly and appeal to our loved ones' senses are some of the most important tricks in a caregiver's bag!

The recipes that follow will help you get through most of the mealtime challenges you'll face. In fact, many will become favorite healthy treats for making precious new memories and indulging your loved one again and again.

Easy Coconut Oatmeal

Here is a really quick breakfast or soft-food meal that takes on any flavor that strikes your fancy: sweet dried fruits, cinnamon, cacao nibs—the sky is the limit!

Yield:	Prep time:	Cook time:	Serving size:
1 cup	30 seconds	1 to 1½ minutes	1 cup

Each serving has:			
32.8 g carbohydrate	15 g fat	3.4 g fiber	4.2 g protein
15 g coconut oil = 1 TB.			

⅓ cup old-fashioned rolled oats

⅔ cup water

Small handful raisins or dried fruit of choice

1 TB. virgin coconut oil

Dash cinnamon (optional)

1. Place old-fashioned rolled oats into a microwavable bowl, along with water, raisins, and virgin coconut oil.

2. Microwave on high power for 1 to 1½ minutes.

3. Stir, sprinkle with cinnamon (if using), and serve.

4. Pat yourself on the back because you haven't even dirtied a pot!

TROPICAL TIP

The first few times, watch the bowl carefully so that it doesn't overflow. Different microwave ovens, the type of bowl you use, and variations in water temperature will dictate exactly the right amount of cooking time.

If it turns out that the oats are not sweet enough, try a different fruit or add a teaspoon of sugar or honey. Over time, you can eliminate the added sugar by reducing it slightly week by week, and no one will ever be the wiser.

Healthy "Anytime Smoothies"

The soothing essences of vanilla, almond, and coconut come together to delight, nourish, and satisfy—even at a moment's notice.

Yield:	Prep time:	Serving size:
2 cups	3 minutes	2 cups

Each serving has:			
16 g carbohydrate	64 g fat	8 g fiber	8 g protein
5.33 g coconut oil = .36 TB.			

1 (14-oz.) can coconut milk	¼ tsp. almond extract
2 TB. whey protein powder	1 tsp. Manuka honey
1 TB. virgin coconut oil	(optional)
1 TB. ground flaxseed	8 ice cubes
1 tsp. organic vanilla extract	

1. Place coconut milk, whey protein powder, virgin coconut oil, ground flaxseed, organic vanilla extract, almond extract, and Manuka honey (if using) in a blender.

2. Blend at high speed until well combined.

3. Stop the blender, add ice cubes, and process again until ice has been incorporated. Serve immediately.

Variation: While predictable routines are comforting to dementia patients, Anytime Smoothies need never become boring. Keep things interesting by tossing in some frozen or fresh seasonal fruit. Items to consider include berries, banana, and avocado.

TO YOUR HEALTH!

Know someone who's crazy for chocolate? Blend in a spoonful of cacao nibs. Cacao is one of the healthiest foods on earth. Unlike processed dark chocolate, antioxidants are preserved in raw cacao. Among other benefits, cacao's antioxidants have been clinically proven to dissolve plaque buildup in the arteries, helping to reverse heart disease and naturally lower blood pressure.

Grilled Pineapple and Mahogany Sticky Rice

The flavors and tropical scents of grilled pineapple, cardamom, and coconut are infused into this warm Southeast Asian dessert salad.

Yield:	Prep time:	Cook time:	Serving size:
3 cups pineapple and 3 cups rice	5 minutes	1 hour	½ cup pineapple and ½ cup rice

Each serving has:			
44 g carbohydrate	6 g fat	3 g fiber	5 g protein
5.33 g coconut oil = .36 TB.			

1 cup uncooked mahogany or black japonica rice	3 TB. packed brown sugar
2 cups water	½ tsp. salt
1 TB. virgin coconut oil	1 medium ripe pineapple, peeled and cut into ½-in. rounds
1 (14-oz.) can coconut milk	
½ tsp. cardamom	

1. Measure uncooked mahogany rice, water, and virgin coconut oil into a medium saucepan. (Choose a saucepan with a lid.) Bring water to a boil over medium-high heat. Reduce heat to low.

2. Cover saucepan, and allow rice to steam until all water has been absorbed, about 30 minutes. Rice grains should be firm but not hard.

3. In a separate medium saucepan, bring coconut milk to a boil, reduce heat to medium-low, and stir in cardamom, brown sugar, and salt until completely dissolved.

4. Remove about ⅔ cup of spiced coconut milk and set aside.

5. Stir rice into the saucepan with spiced coconut milk. Bring milk to a simmer, cover, and cook for about 20 minutes more, until liquid is absorbed.

6. While rice is simmering, heat and oil a grill or grill plate.

7. When the grill is hot, grill pineapple rounds about 2 minutes per side or until slightly charred and tender.

8. Remove pineapple rounds from the grill. When cool enough to handle, dice pineapple into bite-size pieces.

9. Serve rice topped with warm pineapple chunks and drizzled with reserved spiced coconut milk.

Variation: This dish is delicious using grilled fresh mango or banana as a substitute for the pineapple. Medium-grain white rice can also be used instead of the mahogany or black rice, but it will yield a dish that provides less fiber—which can be a serious consideration when cooking for elderly dementia patients. Cooking times for white rice will need to be reduced.

TROPICAL TIP

While this dish is reminiscent of rice pudding, mahogany and black rice will always remain a little bit chewy when done.

Yummy Coconut Macaroons

These delightful macaroons are not overly sweet, giving center stage to the real flavor of coconut.

Yield:	Prep time:	Cook time:	Serving size:
1 dozen cookies	5 minutes	15 minutes	2 cookies

Each serving has:			
3.8 g carbohydrate	9.6 g fat	1.2 g fiber	2.7 g protein
4 g coconut oil = .27 TB.			

2 TB. warm water

1 TB. Manuka honey

1 cup unsweetened coconut flakes

1 whole large egg, beaten

1. Preheat the oven to 400°F.

2. In a medium bowl, mix warm water and Manuka honey together.

3. Add unsweetened coconut flakes and beaten egg. Stir until thoroughly combined.

4. Form mixture into tablespoon-size balls and drop by the spoonful onto a well-greased cookie sheet.

5. Bake at 400°F for 12 to 15 minutes. Cookies will slightly singe in spots but will not brown.

6. Allow to cool 3 to 5 minutes before transferring to serve.

TO YOUR HEALTH!

These coconut macaroons are soft and chewy and oh-so-comforting. They are also far healthier than cookie recipes that call for flour, salt, and other dubious ingredients—and they're gluten free, too! When you have a real craving for a taste of something sweet, these macaroons offer a truly healthy choice.

Chocolate Coconut Pudding

Even people who don't like coconut will love this richly flavorful, nutty chocolate pudding.

Yield:	Prep time:	Serving size:	
½ cup	5 minutes	¼ cup	
Each serving has:			
58.1 g carbohydrate	18.5 g fat	4 g fiber	2.6 g protein
2.9 g coconut oil = .19 TB.			

4 TB. unsweetened cocoa powder

6 TB. Manuka honey

2 TB. water

2 tsp. coconut cream concentrate (also known as coconut butter)

2 tsp. virgin coconut oil

1 TB. coarsely chopped pecans

1. In a small mixing bowl, combine unsweetened cocoa powder, Manuka honey, water, coconut cream concentrate, virgin coconut oil, and chopped pecans.

2. Mix until thoroughly combined.

3. Serve in a small desert bowl at room temperature.

Variation: To make **Chocolate Coconut Fudge,** double or triple the pudding recipe's amounts and combine the ingredients. Line a square cake pan or loaf pan with a sheet of waxed paper. Smooth mixture into the pan and chill in the refrigerator. When firm, cut into squares and serve.

TROPICAL TIP

Warming the coconut cream concentrate, honey, and coconut oil will help make them easier to measure and will aid in combining the ingredients.

Coconut Parfait

Icy cold coconut parfait delights the palate with crisp orange notes and sumptuous freshly whipped cream.

Yield:	Prep time:	Cook time:	Serving size:
6 parfaits	1 hour	5 minutes	¾ cup
Each serving has:			
27.1 g carbohydrate 16.3 g fat		2.4 g fiber	1.3 g protein
8 g coconut oil = .53 TB.			

Several drops red food coloring (optional)

1 cup heavy whipping cream

1⅓ cups water

⅔ cup granulated sugar

1 TB. orange extract

2 cups grated young coconut

6 sprigs fresh mint

1. Add enough food coloring (if using) to whipping cream to tint it a deep pink color.

2. Using a hand mixer or wire whisk and a medium mixing bowl, whip cream until soft peaks form. Set aside.

3. In a medium saucepan, make a simple syrup by boiling water and sugar together for 3 to 5 minutes. Pour into a heatproof glass dish to cool.

4. Stir orange extract into cooled simple syrup. Add coconut and whipped cream, stirring until well combined, and place in the freezer. Freeze until mixture is a semifirm slush. Begin checking after 30 minutes.

5. Remove from the freezer and beat mixture with a wire whisk until frothy.

6. Fill parfait glasses with mixture and freeze until firm. Serve cold, garnished with a sprig of fresh mint.

TROPICAL TIP

You can substitute 1½ cups packaged dry flaked coconut for the grated young coconut. If you're using packaged coconut, allow the coconut to soak in ½ cup of milk for 30 minutes. Then drain the milk away from the soaked coconut before using in the recipe. If you reserve the drained milk, it can do double duty as a flavoring for coffee or breakfast cereal.

Coconut Pudding (Haupia)

The pure and unadulterated flavor of native coconut, as found in traditional Hawaiian haupia, is a dish without which no luau would be complete.

Yield:	Prep time:	Cook time:	Serving size:
6 squares (3 cups)	3 minutes	30 minutes	1 (½-cup) square

Each serving has:			
18.6 g carbohydrate	4 g fat	2.7 g fiber	2.8 g protein
8.5 g coconut oil = .57 TB.			

3 cups coconut milk	¼ tsp. vanilla extract
4 TB. granulated sugar	3 TB. cornstarch
Dash salt	

1. In a medium saucepan, heat 2¾ cups coconut milk over medium-low heat—do not allow it to boil.

2. Stir in sugar, salt, and vanilla extract to combine.

3. Mix remaining ¼ cup coconut milk with cornstarch and add gradually to the saucepan, stirring until mixture thickens. Haupia will form a skin on the surface of a cooling spoon when it has thickened enough.

4. Pour haupia into a square cake pan. Refrigerate until set.

5. Cut into 6 even portions and serve chilled.

Variation: Chill haupia in beautiful individual molds and unmold onto pretty dessert plates. Serve decorated with tinted or toasted flaked coconut and a spoon of fruit compote on the side.

TROPICAL TIP

At a traditional luau, this glistening white coconut pudding is sliced into small cubes and served on fresh ti leaves.

Island Custard

The flavors of almond and maraschino cherries define this velvety smooth, meringue-topped custard.

Yield:	Prep time:	Cook time:	Serving size:
6 custard cups	10 minutes	20 minutes	1 custard cup

Each serving has:			
41 g carbohydrate	10.2 g fat	2.1 g fiber	7.7 g protein
2.8 g coconut oil = .19 TB.			

2 cups milk	1 tsp. almond extract
1 (3½-oz.) can flaked coconut	10 maraschino cherries, chopped
4 egg yolks, beaten	
⅛ tsp. salt	4 egg whites
¾ cup granulated sugar	6 whole maraschino cherries

1. Combine milk and coconut in a medium saucepan over low heat. Cook, stirring occasionally, for 5 minutes.

2. Using a double boiler and mixing well, combine egg yolks, salt, and ¼ cup sugar over boiling water.

3. Gradually add milk and coconut mixture and cook, stirring constantly, until mixture coats the spoon when lifted from the pot.

4. Remove from heat, stir in almond extract and cool for 3 to 5 minutes.

5. Spoon into dessert cups or parfait glasses and chill.

6. Sprinkle the top of each dessert cup with chopped cherries.

7. With a wire whisk or hand mixer, beat egg whites until very foamy but not too stiff.

8. Gradually begin adding remaining ½ cup sugar while continuing to beat egg whites, until all sugar has been incorporated and whites are stiff and glossy.

9. Top each custard cup with a mound of beaten egg whites, garnish each meringue with 1 whole maraschino cherry, and serve.

> **TROPICAL TIP**
>
> Egg white meringues can be temperamental little creations, but don't fret! Here are some tips:
>
> - Egg whites are easiest to separate when they are cold—straight from the refrigerator.
> - Allow egg whites to come to room temperature before you begin beating them.
> - Egg whites and the utensils you use must be very clean. Do not allow a speck of fat or egg yolk to come in contact with the egg whites, bowl, or whisk.

Coconut Mousse Pie

This pie is a delicately sweet dessert perfect for special occasions.

Yield:	Prep time:	Serving size:	
1 9-inch pie	30 minutes	1 wedge (⅛ pie)	
Each serving has:			
19 g carbohydrate	40.8 g fat	2.7 g fiber	6.6 g protein
13.25 g coconut oil = .88 TB.			

4 egg yolks	4 egg whites
½ cup granulated sugar	Pinch salt
1 tsp. vanilla extract	1 cup finely shredded, dried, unsweetened coconut
1 tsp. coconut extract	
1 cup heavy cream	1 baked Coconut Piecrust (see next recipe)
1 TB. unflavored gelatin, dissolved in 2 TB. water	2 cups whipped cream

1. In a medium mixing bowl, beat egg yolks and sugar together until mixture forms a pale ribbon when the beater is lifted from the bowl.

2. Stir in vanilla extract, coconut extract, heavy cream, and gelatin.

3. In a separate bowl, beat egg whites with salt until stiff peaks form.

4. Gently fold egg yolk mixture and shredded coconut into beaten egg whites to create mousse.

5. Fill baked piecrust with mousse and chill well.

6. When pie is fully chilled, top with whipped cream, cut into 8 wedges, and serve.

TO YOUR HEALTH!

Scientists have described over 60 species of coconut palm. Today, however, there is only one species, nucifera. Within this species are over 80 varieties of coconut palm that are loosely grouped according to whether they are tall or dwarf varieties.

Coconut Piecrust

This piecrust is a delicious and unusual way to introduce even more coconut goodness into your diet and pairs well with the Coconut Mousse Pie recipe.

Yield:	Prep time:	Cooking time:	Serving size:
1 9-inch piecrust	5 minutes	30 minutes	1 wedge (⅛ crust)

Each serving has:			
3 g carbohydrate	36 g fat	1.8 g fiber	.7 g protein
36 g coconut oil = 2.4 TB.			

½ cup coconut oil

2 cups unsweetened flaked coconut

1. Mix ½ cup coconut oil and 2 cups unsweetened flaked coconut in a small bowl.

2. Press mixture into a 9-inch pie plate.

3. Bake at 300°F for 30 minutes or until deeply golden.

4. Allow to cool completely before filling.

Chewy Peanut Butter Coconut Granola Bars

For fun snacking or an easy make-ahead breakfast, the chewy, peanutty goodness of these granola bars can't be beat.

Yield:	Prep time:	Cook time:	Serving size:
12 granola bars	10 minutes	25 minutes	1 granola bar

Each serving has:			
60 g carbohydrate	13.7 g fat	7 g fiber	8.9 g protein
6 g coconut oil = .4 TB.			

1 cup *rapadura* or sugar	⅓ cup coconut flour
½ cup Manuka honey	½ cup flaked coconut
⅔ cup peanut butter	½ cup sunflower seeds
½ cup (1 stick) unsalted butter, melted	½ cup raisins
2 tsp. vanilla extract	½ cup chocolate chips (optional)
3 cups rolled oats	

1. Preheat the oven to 350°F. In a large mixing bowl, combine rapadura, Manuka honey, peanut butter, unsalted butter, and vanilla extract. Stir together until well combined.

2. Stir in rolled oats, coconut flour, flaked coconut, sunflower seeds, raisins, and chocolate chips (if using). Mixture will resemble a damp granola cereal.

3. Press evenly into a greased jellyroll pan or glass baking dish. Bake 25 minutes or until edges are brown.

4. Remove from the oven. While still warm, use a butter knife to cut baked mixture into bars and slide the knife around the edges of the pan to loosen. Allow to cool and firm completely before handling.

5. Remove bars from the pan and serve. Store any leftover bars in an airtight container in the refrigerator for handy snacking.

> **DEFINITION**
>
> **Rapadura** (also called jaggery) is a commercial name for dehydrated cane sugar juice that the people of India have used for thousands of years. Unlike the empty calories of table sugar, rapadura is a rich source of minerals—especially silica—and is a good substitute for sugar in cookies and cakes.

Samoan Bananas with Coconut Sauce (Toifa'l)

Here's a warm desert for using up your flavorful, very-ripe bananas before they're too far gone.

Yield:	Prep time:	Cook time:	Serving size:
6 bananas	10 minutes	30 minutes	1 banana

Each serving has:			
30.6 g carbohydrate 11.5 g fat		3.8 g fiber	1.9 g protein
9 g coconut oil = .6 TB.			

6 small ripe bananas, peeled and cut into 1-in. chunks	1 cup heavy cream
2 TB. coconut oil	2 TB. granulated sugar
1 cup unsweetened flaked coconut	Whipped cream
	6 maraschino cherries

1. In a large skillet, sauté bananas in coconut oil until soft and keep hot in a warm oven.

2. Combine unsweetened flaked coconut, heavy cream, and sugar in a saucepan and simmer over medium heat for 15 to 20 minutes.

3. Divide banana chunks equally into 6 dessert bowls.

4. Pour sauce over bananas.

5. Top with whipped cream and a maraschino cherry. Serve warm.

Samoan Papaya Dessert

Juicy, ripe papaya and coconut come together to produce a bright-tasting, chilly dessert.

Yield:	Prep time:	Serving size:	
3 cups	10 minutes	½ cup	
Each serving has:			
7.1 g carbohydrate	9.6 g fat	1.7 g fiber	1.2 g protein
9.5 g coconut oil = .64 TB.			

2 very ripe small papayas, peeled and seeded (about 2 cups)	1 TB. lemon or lime juice
	1 cup coconut cream
1 tsp. salt	Flaked coconut
1 (¼ in. thick) slice ginger root, minced	6 maraschino cherries

1. Using a blender, purée papayas along with salt, ginger root, lemon juice, and coconut cream. Blend until well combined.

2. Spoon into parfait glasses and chill.

3. Sprinkle with flaked coconut, top with a maraschino cherry, and serve cold.

Homemade Hygiene, Hair, and Skin-Care Products

In This Chapter

- Your internal mirror
- Nutrition from the outside in
- Natural nurture and protection of the body
- Personal-care products to make and use

The skin is the largest organ of the body. It is the vital protective covering for our body, without which we could not live. Through perspiration and evaporation, the skin also functions as an important means of toxin elimination. Because skin grows rapidly and its cells are constantly being replaced, it has an intense requirement for nourishment.

As an intermediary between our internal and external environments, the skin is able to reflect how the internal systems of the body are functioning. Firm, smooth, dewy skin bespeaks a condition of youthfulness and health that is universally recognized. Dry, flakey, puffy, or inflamed skin indicates there is something awry internally.

By the same token, however, the skin acts as a sponge or an organ of uptake. While drinking adequate amounts of water and eating wholesome foods are necessary for overall health and therefore the health of the skin, the skin, by its ability to absorb both nutrients and toxins, ultimately affects the health of the internal body. It is a two-way street.

TO YOUR HEALTH!

Have you ever read the back of your shampoo bottle? The ingredients read something like this:

Ammonium laureth sulfate, ammonium lauryl sulfate, cocamidopropyl betaine, ammonium chloride, disodium laureth sulfosuccinate, fragrance, hydroxypropyl methylcellulose, disodium EDTA, methylchloroisothiazolinone, benzophenone-4, citric acid, propylene glycol, triethylene glycol, tetrasodium EDTA, benzyl alcohol, methylsothiazolinone, benzyl benzoate, butylphenyl methylpropional, Red 40 (CI 16035), Ext. Violet 2 (CI60730), Redd 33 (CI17200), Blue 1 (CI 42090), and Yellow 5 (CI 19140).

Nutritionists tell us not to eat foods with ingredients we cannot pronounce. So why allow your skin to absorb chemicals that you wouldn't eat?

Natural Products Are Better

Healthy care of one's skin, hair, and personal hygiene using cleansers, moisturizers, and beauty products means finding the fine line between nurture and excessive exposure to toxic chemicals. For example:

- Modern deodorants contain aluminum salts like aluminum chlorohydrate, and aluminum has been strongly associated with neurodegenerative diseases such as Alzheimer's.

- Commercially available toothpastes contain fluoride, which is a toxic by-product of the aluminum manufacturing industry.

- Body washes and shampoos contain sodium lauryl sulfate, a surfactant found in engine degreasers that not only causes irritation but also denatures skin proteins, allowing environmental contaminants easier access to the deep, sensitive layers of the skin.

- Sunscreens block the skin's ability to produce vitamin D, a vital hormone that protects against cancer, osteoporosis, osteomalacia, multiple sclerosis, and depression. Simultaneously, sunscreens expose the skin to oxybenzone, a chemical that has been linked to allergies, hormone disruption, and cell damage.

Overall, natural skin-nurturing products are a safer alternative for self-care, and they don't carry the danger of chronic toxic chemical exposure. Aloe vera products, clay packs, herbal wraps, essential oils, and honey are a few options for safely cleaning, detoxifying, and nurturing our skin, and coconut oil provides its own unique nurturing properties to add to the mix.

AW, NUTS!

Take care when selecting essential oils. *Essential* oils and *fragrance* oils are not the same thing. Essential oils are natural compounds that have been distilled from the leaves, flowers, stems, roots, or bark of plants. Many are used medicinally for their health-giving properties. Fragrance oils are synthetically manufactured chemical compounds that imitate the fragrance attributes of a plant's volatile oils, but they have no known health-giving properties and may be very toxic to the body. See Appendix B for product sources for essential oils.

In this chapter, you will discover natural methods for creating many of your own personal-care products based on the health-promoting qualities of coconut oil, high-grade essential oils, and other wholesome natural products.

Coconut Toothpaste

Homemade coconut oil toothpaste will not foam because it does not contain harsh ingredients like sodium lauryl sulfate, but it will leave your mouth wonderfully fresh and minty clean.

3 TB. coconut oil

3 TB. baking soda

¼ tsp. (25 drops) peppermint essential oil

1 packet stevia powder (optional)

2 tsp. glycerin (optional)

1. Place coconut oil and baking soda in a small bowl. Stir them together until well blended. (A mortar and pestle work very well for this.)

2. By carefully counting each drop or using a standard measuring spoon, add peppermint essential oil to mixture.

3. Add stevia powder (if using) and glycerin (if using) and stir well to combine.

4. This dentifrice can be thinned to your taste using distilled water.

5. Store in a clean jar for use as needed. Apply to a clean, dry toothbrush. Brush teeth and rinse mouth as usual.

Variation: If your teeth or gums are sensitive, try adding 5 drops of clove oil along with the peppermint oil. Clove oil is a good antiseptic and effectively numbs pain.

AW, NUTS!

Essential oils are very powerful substances and should be treated with respect. Each drop of the highly concentrated plant extract is equivalent to at least 1 ounce of whole plant material. Therefore, it is wise to respect established formula recommendations and dosages.

Homemade Underarm Deodorant

This recipe makes a lavender-scented, cream-style deodorant. In cool climates, it can be stored in a clean, empty stick-deodorant dispenser.

2 TB. coconut oil	5 TB. arrowroot or cornstarch
⅛ tsp. (13 drops) lavender essential oil	3 TB. baking soda

1. Place coconut oil and lavender essential oil in a small bowl. Stir well to combine.

2. Add arrowroot and baking soda to oil mixture and thoroughly combine. You should not see any dry ingredients or globs of unincorporated coconut oil.

3. Store mixture in a covered jar. Store the filled deodorant dispenser in the refrigerator overnight to allow it to properly set.

4. Lightly apply using fingertips.

TROPICAL TIP

Very little of this deodorant is required, so apply it lightly. Coconut oil and lavender essential oil both have antibacterial properties, which make them highly effective at preventing odor.

Soothing Herbal Deodorant

The same soothing, therapeutic qualities of chamomile and catnip teas effuse their calming essences through the skin.

3 TB. loose chamomile tea	3 TB. baking soda
2 TB. loose catnip tea	6 TB. arrowroot (or cornstarch)
5 TB. coconut oil, melted	¼ tsp. (25 drops) tea tree oil
3 TB. apricot kernel oil	

1. In a dry, sterilized jar, place chamomile tea, catnip tea, coconut oil, and apricot kernel oil. Cover tightly and shake well.

2. Place the jar in a warm but dark place to infuse for 2 to 3 weeks. (A cabinet over the stove or refrigerator may be ideal.) Shake the jar once every other day.

3. In a shallow pan of water, gently warm the jar of oil to ensure that it is completely liquefied.

4. Using a sieve, strain warm oil into a medium bowl. Add baking soda, arrowroot, and tea tree oil. Stir well to combine.

5. Store deodorant in a sealed, sterilized jar and use as usual to prevent underarm odor.

TO YOUR HEALTH!

Chamomile and catnip are herbs that have impressive calming properties. Infusions applied to the skin relieve inflammation.

Coconut Lip Balm

Protect your lips from harsh winter winds and hot summer sun with nourishing, fun-to-make, homemade coconut oil lip balm.

½ cup almond oil

¼ cup cocoa butter (or shea butter)

¼ cup coconut oil

1 TB. honey

¼ cup (2 oz.) beeswax

1½ tsp. natural extract of choice (vanilla, cherry, orange, etc.)

1. In a small saucepan, mix together almond oil, cocoa butter, and coconut oil over low heat.

2. Stir in honey and beeswax. Continue stirring until completely melted.

3. Stir in naturally flavored extract. Spoon a small amount onto a heatproof plate and allow to cool.

4. Test for firmness. If the cooled lip balm is not firm, add a bit more beeswax to the saucepan. Melt while stirring and test again.

5. Pour finished lip balm into handy-size small tins or jars and allow to cool completely.

TROPICAL TIP

Make several batches of coconut oil lip balm in a variety of flavors. They make wonderfully thoughtful gifts!

Coconut Oil as a Mouthwash

Straight coconut oil can be used as a mouth rinse to enhance oral health, as practiced in traditional Ayurvedic medicine.

1 to 3 tsp. coconut oil

1. Brush teeth as usual. Rinse mouth.

2. Place 1 to 3 teaspoons coconut oil in mouth (as much as is comfortable) and purse lips tightly. Push, pull, and swish oil around the mouth and between teeth for 15 to 20 minutes. (This is not a misprint.) You can do this while you make your coffee, blow your hair dry, or even while you shower.

3. Spit oil out into the sink.

> **TO YOUR HEALTH!**
>
> In Dr. Bruce Fife's excellent book *Oil Pulling Therapy,* he explains how to implement this ancient method of healing and detoxifying the body through oral hygiene. If you have an active oral infection, he recommends adding a drop of clove or oregano oil and the contents of a CoQ10 capsule to the coconut oil before swishing.

Sunscreen and After-Sun Moisturizer

Coconut oil, all by itself, will make an excellent skin protectant and nourishing moisturizer. But these recipes will afford your skin some added protection and nurturing.

Sunscreen:

⅓ cup coconut oil

¼ cup 100 percent aloe vera gel

4 tsp. titanium dioxide

1 TB. zinc oxide

1. In a double boiler over gentle heat, melt coconut oil.

2. Remove from heat and stir in aloe vera gel.

3. Stir in titanium dioxide and zinc oxide to thoroughly combine.

4. Apply and reapply as necessary—this sunscreen is not waterproof.

5. Store in a plastic container in the refrigerator when not in use.

After-Sun Moisturizer:

¼ cup coconut oil

½ cup 100 percent aloe vera gel

2 tsp. (100 drops) lavender essential oil

1. In a double boiler over gentle heat, melt coconut oil.

2. Remove from heat and stir in aloe vera gel.

3. Stir in lavender essential oil to combine.

TO YOUR HEALTH!

Lavender essential oil helps to take the sting out of wind-, sun-, or chlorine-damaged skin.

Hair Conditioner for Deep Conditioning

This is an excellent method for deeply conditioning your hair. Just be sure you have an hour or two of time to devote to the process before you begin.

1 tsp. coconut oil

1. Apply coconut oil to hair, beginning at the scalp and working it all the way down to the ends.

2. Gently massage scalp.

3. Comb through entire length of hair.

4. Wrap hair in a hot, damp towel and set the timer for 1 to 2 hours.

5. When the timer rings, remove the towel and wash hair as usual. It may take more than one washing to remove all of the excess oil.

6. Do not condition. Rinse and style as usual.

> **TROPICAL TIP**
>
> Does your hair suffer from frizzies? Kiss them good-bye today: Rub a pea-size dab of coconut oil (smaller if you have short hair) between the palms of your hands. Run your fingers through dry hair and scrunch or comb through as usual.

Moisturizing Body Butter

This luxurious body butter immediately begins to repair, moisturize, and soften skin.

1 cup shea butter
½ cup coconut oil
½ cup almond oil

½ tsp. (50 drops) lavender essential oil

1. In the top of a double boiler, gently melt shea butter and coconut oil.

2. Set aside and allow to cool for 30 minutes.

3. Stir in almond oil and lavender essential oil. Set aside.

4. When oils have become opaque and nearly solid, use a hand mixer or balloon whisk to beat the oils until a whipped butter consistency is achieved.

5. Store, covered, in a clean glass jar.

> **TROPICAL TIP**
>
> A surprisingly tiny amount of body butter will cover a large area of skin. Apply sparingly at first and massage into skin until completely absorbed.

Intimate Body Balm

Chocolate lovers will fall head over heels for this body balm—it's so good, you'll be tempted to eat it!

3 TB. almond oil

2 TB. cocoa butter

1 TB. food-grade glycerin

2 tsp. beeswax, grated and firmly packed

2 tsp. unsweetened cocoa powder

2 tsp. honey

⅛ tsp. (13 drops) cinnamon essential oil

1. In the top of a double boiler, gently heat and stir together almond oil, cocoa butter, glycerin, and beeswax until beeswax is completely melted. Remove from heat.

2. While still warm, beat in cocoa powder, honey, and cinnamon essential oil using a small wire whisk.

3. Store, covered, in a clean small container.

4. Allow to cool completely before using.

AW, NUTS!

While this is a fun and delicious way to share the health benefits of coconut oil with your most significant other, be forewarned—this body balm will damage latex! Rubber and coconut oil do not mix.

Test a small amount on the inside of your wrist or elbow for 24 hours before using. Cinnamon oil can be an irritant to some, and chocolate is a common allergen.

Glossary

acrylamide A substance formed in heated oils that is known to cause cancer in animals and nerve damage in humans. Industrially, it is used in the manufacture of dyes, plastics, caulking, food packaging, and some adhesives.

Activator X Vitamin K_2, first described by Weston A. Price, DDS. It was once thought that the benefits of vitamin K were limited to its role in blood clotting and that vitamins K_1 and K_2 were simply different forms of the same vitamin and possessed the same physiological functions. It is now known that the benefits of vitamin K_2 include, among other things, promotion of bone, cardiovascular, skin, brain, and prostate health.

activity-induced thermogenesis Heat energy fueled by the calories burned in any activity, such as housekeeping, walking, or riding a bicycle.

adipose tissue A type of body tissue that contains stored cellular fat, serves as a source of energy, cushions and insulates vital organs, and is active in the formation of hormones.

aioli A classic French sauce originating from the cuisine of Provence, where it is usually served as a condiment with meat, fish, cooked vegetables, or crudités.

all-purpose flour Flour that contains only the inner part of the wheat grain. Usable for all purposes from cakes to gravies.

amino acids The building blocks from which proteins are made.

anaerobic respiration A form of cellular respiration that occurs when oxygen is scarce or absent.

antioxidant A substance that reduces damaging oxidation caused by free radicals. Well-known antioxidants include vitamins C and E. Antioxidants reduce the risk of cancer and the development of age-related diseases.

Ayurvedic medicine (also **Ayurveda**) One of the world's oldest medical systems. It was developed in India and has evolved over thousands of years. The term "Ayurveda" is comprised of the Sanskrit words *ayur* (life) and *veda* (science or knowledge)—literally meaning, "the science of life." In the West, Ayurvedic medicine is considered a complementary medical system because it evolved apart from modern allopathic medicine. Ayurveda employs the use of herbs and specially tailored diets and techniques designed to balance the body, mind, and spirit.

bake To cook in a dry oven. Dry-heat cooking often results in a crisping of the exterior of the food being cooked. Moist-heat cooking, through methods such as steaming, poaching, etc., brings a much different, moist quality to the food.

bamboo shoots Crunchy, tasty, white parts of the growing bamboo plant, often purchased canned.

basal metabolic rate The rate at which calories are used up in the regulation of normal bodily functions—while sleeping, for example.

basil A flavorful, almost sweet, resinous herb that is delicious with tomatoes and used in all kinds of Italian or Mediterranean-style dishes.

baste To keep foods moist during cooking by spooning, brushing, or drizzling with a liquid.

beat To quickly mix substances.

bioflavonoids Once known as vitamin P, these are classes of plant metabolites found in the natural pigments in fruits and vegetables. Three of the flavonoid classes are ketone-containing compounds that show much promise in preventing and mitigating neurodegenerative disease states such as the various dementias, MS, ALS, and Parkinson's disease.

bilayer The self-aligning structure that forms the interior and exterior boundary of a cell. It is made up of pairs of phospholipids that have a hydrophobic tail and hydrophilic head.

blend   To completely mix something, usually with a blender or food processor, more slowly than beating.

body mass index (BMI)   A relative measure of ideal weight determined by using one of the following two formulas: *English:* BMI = [weight in pounds ÷ (height in inches)^2]× 703; *Metric:* BMI = weight in kilograms ÷ (height in meters)^2

boil   To heat a liquid to a point where water is forced to turn into steam, causing the liquid to bubble. To boil something is to insert it into boiling water. A rapid boil is when a lot of bubbles rise to the surface of the liquid.

bok choy (also **Chinese cabbage**)   A member of the cabbage family with thick stems, crisp texture, and fresh flavor. It's perfect for stir-frying.

brine   A highly salted, often seasoned, liquid used to flavor and preserve foods. To brine a food is to soak, or preserve, it by submerging it in brine. The salt in the brine penetrates the fibers of the meat and makes it moist and tender.

broth   *See* stock.

brown   To cook in a skillet, turning, until the food's surface is seared and brown in color, to lock in the juices.

brown rice   Whole-grain rice including the germ, with a characteristic pale brown or tan color; more nutritious and flavorful than white rice.

buko juice   The clear liquid (coconut water) inside young coconuts. It is a very popular drink in the tropics, especially in Southeast Asia, the Pacific Islands, Africa, and the Caribbean. Lately it has become available canned or bottled and is now being marketed as a natural sports drink due to its healthy, high-mineral content.

cachexia   A syndrome of progressive weight loss, anorexia, and loss of muscle and body mass. It is often seen in cancer patients as a response to a malignant growth.

carbohydrate   A nutritional component found in starches, sugars, fruits, and vegetables that causes a rise in blood-glucose levels. Carbohydrates supply energy and many important nutrients, including vitamins, minerals, and antioxidants.

cardamom   An intense, sweet-smelling spice, common to Indian cooking and used in baking and coffee.

carob   A tropical tree that produces long pods. The dried, baked, and powdered flesh (carob powder) is used in baking, and the fresh and dried pods are used for a variety of recipes. The flavor is sweet and reminiscent of chocolate.

cayenne   A fiery spice made from (hot) chile peppers, especially the cayenne chile, a slender, red, and very hot pepper.

cerebral hemisphere   One of the halves of the cerebrum. The left and right cerebral hemispheres are divided by a deep fissure and are connected at the base by the corpus callosum. The hemispheres are made up of an external gray layer (the cerebral cortex) and an internal white matter that surrounds gray matter called nuclei (the basal ganglia).

ceviche   Pronounced *suh-vee-chay*. A seafood dish in which fresh fish or seafood is marinated for several hours in highly acidic lemon or lime juice, tomato, onion, and cilantro. The acid "cooks" the seafood.

chiffonade   A technique for cutting leafy herbs into long fine ribbons. The herbs are stacked together and tightly rolled into a log. Then very thin slices are cut from the roll to produce the fine strips of herb.

chiles   Any one of many different "hot" peppers, ranging in intensity from the relatively mild ancho pepper to the blisteringly hot habanero.

chili powder   A seasoning blend that includes chile pepper, cumin, garlic, and oregano. Proportions vary among different versions, but they all offer a warm, rich flavor.

Chinese five-spice powder   A seasoning blend of cinnamon, anise, ginger, fennel, and pepper.

chives   A member of the onion family, chives grow in bunches of long leaves that resemble tall grass or the green tops of onions and offer a light onion flavor.

chop   To cut into pieces, usually qualified by an adverb such as "coarsely chopped" or by a size measurement such as "chopped into $\frac{1}{2}$-inch pieces." "Finely chopped" is much closer to mince.

cilantro A member of the parsley family used in Mexican cooking (especially salsa) and some Asian dishes. Use in moderation as the flavor can overwhelm. The seed of the cilantro is the spice coriander.

cinnamon A sweet, rich, aromatic spice commonly used in baking or desserts. Cinnamon can also be used for delicious and interesting entrées.

clove A sweet, strong, almost wintergreen-flavored spice used in baking and with meats such as ham.

copra Dried coconut meat. Copra is an important agricultural commodity for many coconut-producing countries. Coconut oil can be extracted from copra, and the coconut cake that remains as a by-product of the oil-extraction process is used as feed for livestock.

coriander A rich, warm, spicy seed used in all types of recipes, from African to South American, from entrées to desserts.

crudités Pronounced *crew-de-tay*. Fresh vegetables served as an appetizer, often together on one tray.

cumin A fiery, smoky-tasting spice popular in Middle Eastern and Indian dishes. Cumin is a seed; ground cumin seed is the most common form used in cooking.

curd A gelatinous substance resulting from coagulated milk used to make cheese. Curd also refers to dishes of similar texture, such as dishes made with egg (lemon curd).

curing A method of preserving uncooked foods, usually meats or fish, by either salting and smoking or pickling.

curry Rich, spicy, Indian-style sauces and the dishes prepared with them. A curry uses curry powder as its base seasoning.

curry powder A ground blend of rich and flavorful spices used as a basis for curry and many other Indian-influenced dishes. Common ingredients include hot pepper, nutmeg, cumin, cinnamon, pepper, and turmeric. Some curry can also be found in paste form.

custard A cooked mixture of eggs and milk, popular as a base for desserts.

dash A few drops, usually of a liquid, released by a quick shake of, for example, a bottle of hot sauce.

deglaze   To scrape up the bits of meat and seasoning left in a pan or skillet after cooking. Usually this is done by adding a liquid such as wine or broth and creating a flavorful stock that can be used to create sauces.

devein   The removal of the dark vein from the back of a large shrimp with a sharp knife.

dice   To cut into small cubes about ¼ inch square.

Dijon mustard   Hearty, spicy mustard made in the style of the Dijon region of France.

dollop   A spoonful of something creamy and thick, like sour cream or whipped cream.

double boiler   A set of two pots designed to nest together, one inside the other, and provide consistent, moist heat for foods that need delicate treatment. The bottom pot holds water (that doesn't quite touch the bottom of the top pot); the top pot holds the ingredient you want to heat.

dredge   To cover a piece of food with a dry substance such as flour or cornmeal.

drizzle   To lightly sprinkle drops of a liquid over food, often as the finishing touch to a dish.

emulsion   A combination of liquid ingredients that do not normally mix well, beaten together to create a thick liquid such as a fat or oil with water. Creation of an emulsion must be done carefully and rapidly to ensure that particles of one ingredient are suspended in the other.

entrée   The main dish in a meal. In France, however, the entrée is considered the first course.

extra-virgin olive oil   *See* olive oil.

fillet   A piece of meat or seafood with the bones removed.

flake   To break into thin sections, as with fish.

floret   The flower or bud end of broccoli or cauliflower.

flour   Grains ground into a meal. Wheat is perhaps the most common flour. Flour is also made from oats, rye, buckwheat, soybeans, etc. *See also* all-purpose flour; whole-wheat flour.

fold   To combine a dense and light mixture with a circular action from the middle of the bowl.

garlic   A member of the onion family that is a pungent and flavorful element in many savory dishes. A garlic bulb contains multiple cloves. Each clove, when chopped, provides about 1 teaspoon garlic. Most recipes call for cloves or chopped garlic by the teaspoon.

garnish   An embellishment not vital to the dish but added to enhance visual appeal.

ginger   Available in fresh root or dried, ground form, ginger adds a pungent, sweet, and spicy quality to a dish.

glycemic index   A relative measure of the rate and level of blood-sugar increase resulting from food consumption.

goiter   The unnatural enlargement of the thyroid gland. This can occur when the thyroid is producing either too much hormone or too little, sometimes even when it is producing the correct amount (called euthyroidism). A goiter indicates that some condition exists that is causing the thyroid gland to grow abnormally.

goitrogens   Substances that suppress the thyroid gland's function by hindering iodine uptake. This can cause a goiter, or an enlargement of the thyroid.

grate   To shave into tiny pieces using a sharp rasp or grater.

grind   To reduce a large, hard substance, often a seasoning such as peppercorns, to the consistency of sand.

handful   An unscientific measurement; the amount of an ingredient you can hold in your hand.

herbes de Provence   A seasoning mix including basil, fennel, marjoram, rosemary, sage, and thyme, common in the south of France.

Herxheimer reactions   A phenomenon originally observed in the treatment of syphilis that has since been described in many other illnesses. The reaction is seen as a temporary increase in symptoms when antibiotics or other substances cause a die-off in the offending pathogen, which, in turn, causes the release of toxins and other debris that the immune system must reject and remove from the body.

hoisin sauce   A sweet Asian condiment similar to ketchup made with soybeans, sesame, chile peppers, and sugar.

hors d'oeuvre   French for "outside of work" (the "work" being the main meal), an hors d'oeuvre can be any dish served as a starter before the meal.

idli   In Indian cuisine, foods that are acidified and leavened by lactic acid bacteria in much the same way sourdough bread is produced, but without the need for wheat or rye proteins. Because of its acidity, the fermentation process protects against food poisoning and the transfer of pathogenic organisms. Because these foods are easily digested, they are often use as food for babies or the infirm.

inflammation   A condition recognized by the presence of heat, pain, reddened tissue, and swelling.

infusion   A liquid in which flavorful ingredients such as herbs have been soaked or steeped to extract that flavor into the liquid.

julienne   A French word meaning "to slice into very thin pieces."

Kalpavriksha (also **Kalpa Vriksha**)   *The Tree of Life*, as recorded in some of the very earliest Sanskrit literature. In some regions of coastal India, this title is accorded to the coconut palm tree.

keratin   A durable protein polymer found only in epithelial cells. It provides the structural strength to the skin, hair, and nails.

keratinocyte   Any one of the cells in the skin that synthesizes keratin.

lentils   Tiny lens-shaped pulses used in European, Middle Eastern, and Indian cuisines.

lipoproteins   Particles that transport lipids (fats) around the body in the blood to where they are needed.

Lp(a) (also **Lipoprotein[a]**)   A subclass of lipoproteins. Numerous genetic and epidemiologic studies have identified Lp(a) as a marker for atherosclerosis, coronary heart disease, and stroke.

malnutrition   The condition that results from adhering to an unbalanced diet, in which certain nutrients are missing, in excess, or in the wrong proportions.

Manuka honey A honey produced in New Zealand by honeybees feeding on the manuka or tea tree. Although the native Maori population has valued it for its healing properties since ancient times for the treatment of internal and external ailments—both serious and minor—recent hospital trials have also shown it to possess amazing antibacterial healing properties.

marinate To soak meat, seafood, or other food in a seasoned sauce, called a marinade, that is high in acid content. The acids break down the muscle of the meat, making it tender and adding flavor.

mastitis A breast infection typically caused by *Staphylococcus aureus*, a common bacteria found on skin. The bacteria enter through an injury or crack in the skin, usually on the nipple. The infection takes place in the fatty tissue of the breast and causes painful swelling and lumps in the infected breast's tissue.

medium-chain triglycerides (MCTs) Six- to twelve-carbon medium-chain fatty acid esters of glycerol. MCTs passively move from the GI tract to the portal vein system without requirement for modification like long-chain fatty acids (more than 12 carbons) or very-long-chain fatty acids (more than 22 carbons).

meld To allow flavors to blend and spread over time. Melding is often why recipes call for overnight refrigeration and is also why some dishes taste better as leftovers.

meringue A baked mixture of sugar and beaten egg whites, often used as a dessert topping.

metabolic syndrome The name for a cluster of risk factors that increases the risk for coronary artery disease, stroke, and type 2 diabetes.

mince To cut into pieces smaller than diced pieces, about $\frac{1}{8}$ inch or smaller.

miso A fermented, flavorful soybean paste, key in many Japanese dishes.

mold A decorative, shaped metal pan in which the contents, such as mousse or gelatin, set up and take the shape of the pan.

monoester   A class of chemical compounds formed by bonding an alcohol and an organic acid, with the loss of one water molecule for each ester group formed. Fats are esters that are produced by bonding fatty acids with the alcohol glycerol.

monolaurin   A monoester formed from lauric acid, which has profound antiviral and antibacterial activity. Since 1966, reports have recognized the antimicrobial activity of the monoglyceride of lauric acid.

moqueca   In the Afro-Brazilian cuisine of Bahia, a regional specialty soup usually made with fresh coconut milk, shrimp, malagueta peppers, and dende oil. Traditionally, it is cooked very slowly over low heat to retain all the vital nutrients of the food.

morbidly obese   People who weigh two or more times their ideal weight and have a BMI of 40 to 49.9. This condition is associated with many serious and life-threatening disorders.

nutmeg   A sweet, fragrant, musky spice used primarily in baking.

NSAID   An acronym for nonsteroidal anti-inflammatory drugs, which are typically used in place of aspirin or corticosteroids to reduce inflammation, pain, and fever. Their generic names include ibuprofen, naproxen, and celecoxib.

obese   People whose body mass index (BMI) is 30 or greater. Obesity results from an abnormal accumulation of body fat and is associated with increased risk of illness, disability, and death.

olive oil   A fragrant liquid produced by crushing or pressing olives. Extra-virgin olive oil—the most flavorful and highest quality—is produced from the first pressing of a batch of olives; oil is also produced from later pressings.

oxidation   The browning of fruit flesh that happens over time and with exposure to air. Minimize oxidation by rubbing the cut surfaces with a lemon half. Oxidation also affects wine, which is why the taste changes over time after a bottle is opened.

Panacea   The goddess of healing in Greek mythology. The daughter of Aesculapius and the sister of Hygeia, Panacea was said to possess a poultice that could cure all disease. Perhaps inspired by the Greek myth, ancient alchemists searched in vain for a *panacea* (lowercase)—a substance that would remedy all sickness and disease.

paprika A rich, red, warm, earthy spice that also lends a rich red color to many dishes.

parsley A fresh-tasting green leafy herb, often used as a garnish.

peppercorns Large, round, dried berries ground to produce pepper.

phenols Chemical compounds found in plants that contain antioxidants that help protect the body against free radical damage and chronic illnesses.

pickle A food, usually a vegetable such as a cucumber, that's been put in brine.

pinch An unscientific measurement term, the amount of an ingredient—typically a dry, granular substance such as an herb or seasoning—you can hold between your finger and thumb.

pita bread A flat, hollow wheat bread often used for sandwiches or sliced pizza-style into slices. Terrific soft with dips or baked or broiled as a vehicle for other ingredients.

poach To cook a food in simmering liquid such as water, wine, or broth.

polyphenols Antioxidants found in certain foods that are believed to also affect cell-to-cell signaling, receptor sensitivity, inflammatory enzyme activity, and gene regulation.

preheat To turn on an oven, broiler, or other cooking appliance in advance of cooking so the temperature will be at the desired level when the assembled dish is ready for cooking.

prostaglandins Naturally occurring fatty acids that act as localized hormones. They stimulate contractility of smooth muscle and the uterus. They have the ability to lower blood pressure and regulate body temperature, blood platelet aggregation, and acid secretion in the stomach. They control inflammation and vascular permeability and affect the action of certain hormones.

purée To reduce a food to a thick, creamy texture, typically using a blender or food processor.

rapadura   The commercial name for dehydrated cane sugar juice that the people of India have used for thousands of years, although in India it is known as jaggery. Unlike the empty calories of table sugar, rapadura is a rich source of minerals—especially silica—and is a good substitute for sugar in cookies and cakes.

reserve   To hold a specified ingredient for another use later in the recipe.

roast   To cook something uncovered in an oven, usually without additional liquid.

roux   A mixture of butter or another fat and flour, used to thicken sauces and soups.

saffron   A spice made from the stamens of crocus flowers, saffron lends a dramatic yellow color and distinctive flavor to a dish. Use only tiny amounts of this expensive herb.

sauté   To pan-cook over lower heat than used for frying.

savory   A popular herb with a fresh, woody taste.

sebum   The oily secretion (made up of keratin, fat, and cellular debris) of the sebaceous glands of the skin. It forms a moist, acidic film that is mildly antifungal and antibacterial and protects the skin and hair against drying.

sesame oil   An oil, made from pressing sesame seeds, that's tasteless if clear and aromatic and flavorful if brown.

shallot   A member of the onion family that grows in a bulb somewhat like garlic and has a milder onion flavor. When a recipe calls for shallot, use the entire bulb.

shellfish   A broad range of seafood, including clams, mussels, oysters, crabs, shrimp, and lobster. Some people are allergic to shellfish, so take care with its inclusion in recipes.

shiitake mushrooms   Large, dark-brown mushrooms with a hearty, meaty flavor. Can be used either fresh or dried, grilled or as a component in other recipes, and as a flavoring source for broth.

short-grain rice   A starchy rice popular for Asian-style dishes because it readily clumps (perfect for eating with chopsticks).

shred   To cut into many long, thin slices.

simmer To boil gently so the liquid barely bubbles.

skillet (also **frying pan**) A generally heavy, flat-bottomed metal pan with a handle designed to cook food over heat on a stovetop or campfire.

skim To remove fat or other material from the top of liquid.

slice To cut into thin pieces.

steam To suspend a food over boiling water and allow the heat of the steam (water vapor) to cook the food. A quick-cooking method, steaming preserves the flavor and texture of a food.

steep To let sit in hot water, as in steeping tea in hot water for 10 minutes.

stew To slowly cook pieces of food submerged in a liquid. Also, a dish that has been prepared by this method.

sticky rice (or **glutinous rice**) *See* short-grain rice.

stir-fry To cook small pieces of food in a wok or skillet over high heat, moving and turning the food quickly to cook all sides.

stock A flavorful broth made by cooking meats and/or vegetables with seasonings until the liquid absorbs these flavors. This liquid is then strained and the solids discarded. It can be eaten alone or used as a base for soups, stews, etc.

tahini A paste made from sesame seeds that is used to flavor many Middle Eastern recipes.

tarragon A sweet, rich-smelling herb perfect with seafood, vegetables (especially asparagus), chicken, and pork.

teriyaki A Japanese-style sauce composed of soy sauce, rice wine, ginger, and sugar that works well with seafood as well as most meats.

thermogenesis The process of metabolic heat production in warm-blooded animals. As a significant component of the metabolic rate, thermogenesis stimulates an increase in energy expenditure and fat oxidation (i.e., fat burning).

toast To heat something, usually bread, so it's browned and crisp.

tofu A cheese-like substance made from soybeans and soy milk.

turmeric   A spicy, pungent, yellow root used in many dishes, especially Indian cuisine, for color and flavor. Turmeric is the source of the yellow color in many prepared mustards.

velouté   One of the five "mother sauces" in classical French cuisine. It serves as a versatile base for many soups and other sauces.

vinegar   An acidic liquid widely used as dressing or seasoning, often made from fermented grapes, apples, or rice. *See also* white vinegar; wine vinegar.

wasabi   Japanese horseradish, a fiery, pungent condiment used with many Japanese-style dishes. Most often sold as a powder, just add water to create a paste.

water chestnuts   A tuber popular in many types of Asian-style cooking. The flesh is white, crunchy, and juicy, and the vegetable holds its texture whether cool or hot.

whey   The liquid milk serum that remains after milk has been curdled and strained—such as in cheese or yogurt making.

whisk   To rapidly mix, introducing air to the mixture.

white vinegar   The most common type of vinegar, produced from grain.

whole-wheat flour   Wheat flour that contains the entire grain.

wild rice   Actually a grass with a rich, nutty flavor, popular as an unusual and nutritious side dish.

wine vinegar   Vinegar produced from red or white wine.

Worcestershire sauce   Originally developed in India and containing tamarind, this spicy sauce is used as a seasoning for many meats and other dishes.

yeast   Tiny fungi that, when mixed with water, sugar, flour, and heat, release carbon dioxide bubbles, which in turn cause the bread to rise.

zest   Small slivers of peel, usually from a citrus fruit such as lemon, lime, or orange.

zester   A kitchen tool used to scrape zest off a fruit. A small grater also works well.

Resources and References

This appendix is provided as a resource for you in your quest to find various foods items and other products that will make your coconut oil diet an enjoyable experience.

It also provides a place from which to launch your own investigations into what coconut oil nutrition and related health research is available, both online and in print.

Food Product Sources

Blair Candy
tinyurl.com/7xl4ltf
Sells coconut snacks and candy.

Coconut Recipes
freecoconutrecipes.com
Provides tons of recipes using coconut products.

Dr. Bernd Friedlander
tinyurl.com/9seh6kb
Sells pharmaceutical-grade MCT Oil.

ImportFood.com
importfood.com
Sells noodles, spices, oils, sauces, and all things Thai.

iShopIndian.com
ishopindian.com
Sells dal (dried lentils), spices, oils, and all things Indian.

Kawaii Aloha, LLC
tinyurl.com/cej63xb
Sells Hawaiian Red Coconut Balls.

Melissa's/World Variety Produce
melissas.com
Sells fresh young coconut, mature coconut, and excellent produce of every kind.

Rockwell Nutrition
rockwellnutrition.com
Sells MCT Colada, a flavorful MCT drink supplement.

Shop West Coast Concessions
tinyurl.com/6rgj45k
Sells Orville "Pour 'N Pop" Popcorn Machine Kits with Coconut Oil.

Tropical Traditions
tropicaltraditions.com
Sells organic virgin and expeller-pressed coconut oil, coconut cream concentrate, flaked coconut, red palm oil, coconut vinegar, coconut flour, organic free-range bison and poultry, raw dairy, and raw Canadian honey.

Young Coconuts
youngcoconuts.com
Sells coconut openers, coconut shredders, coconut de-meaters, coconut scrapers, and the Coconut Noodle Maker.

Hair and Body-Care Product Sources

Jedwards International, Inc.
bulknaturaloils.com
Sells organic and conventional specialty oils, essential oils, butters, waxes, and botanicals.

ProHealth
tiny.cc/jijchw
Sells 50,000 IU vitamin D_3 capsules.

Sedona Aromatherapie
tiny.cc/0zgahw
Sells kits for making your own aromatherapy products.

Tropical Traditions
tropicaltraditions.com
Sells coconut oil–based products, such as tooth cleanser, deodorant, lip balm, hair conditioner, exfoliating cream, hand cream, and face and body balm.

The Vitamin Shoppe
vitaminshoppe.com
Sells essential oils, vitamins, and nutritional supplements.

Further Reading

Atkins, Robert C. *Atkins for Life: The Complete Carb Program for Permanent Weight Loss and Good Health*. New York: St. Martin's Press, 2004.

———. *Dr. Atkins' Age-Defying Diet*. New York: St. Martin's Paperbacks, 2001.

———. *Dr. Atkins' New Diet Revolution*. New York: Avon Books, 1992.

Bowden, Jonny. *The 150 Healthiest Foods on Earth*. Gloucester, MA: Fair Winds Press, 2007.

Calbom, Cherie. *The Coconut Diet*. New York: Warner Books, 2005.

———. *The Ultimate Smoothie Book*. New York: Warner Wellness, 2006.

Daniel, Kaayla T. *The Whole Soy Story*. Washington, D.C.: New Trends Publishing, 2005.

Fallon, Sally, and Mary G. Enig. *Nourishing Traditions*. Washington, D.C.: New Trends Publishing, 2001.

Fife, Bruce. *Oil Pulling Therapy*. Colorado Springs: Piccadilly Books, 2008.

———. *Stop Alzheimer's Now!* Colorado Springs: Piccadilly Books, 2011.

———. *The Coconut Oil Miracle*. New York: Avery, 2004.

Lavabre, Marcel. *Aromatherapy Workbook*. Rochester, VT: Healing Arts Press, 1990.

Mateljan, George. *The World's Healthiest Foods*. Seattle: George Mateljan Foundation, 2007.

Newport, Mary T. *Alzheimer's Disease: What If There Was a Cure?* Laguna Beach, CA: Basic Health Publications, 2011.

O'Brien, John, et al. *Dementia With Lewy Bodies & Parkinson's Disease Dementia*. Boca Raton, FL: Taylor & Francis, 2006. (Recommended for physicians and scientific experts only.)

Parker, James N., and Philip M. Parker. *The Official Patient's Sourcebook on Dementia with Lewy Bodies*. San Diego, CA: ICON Health Publications, 2002.

Price, Weston A. *Nutrition and Physical Degeneration*. La Mesa, CA: "The Price-Pottenger Nutrition Foundation, Inc., 1939.

Shilhavy, Brian, and Marianita Shilhavy. *Virgin Coconut Oil*. West Bend, WI: Tropical Traditions, 2005.

Online Resources

"Beneficial effects of virgin coconut oil on lipid parameters and in vitro LDL oxidation"
tiny.cc/zx99gw
Study by K.G. Nevin and T. Rajamohan, clinical biochemistry.

Blanco Botanicals
blancobotanicals.com
Website of Maria H. Blanco, Certified Family Herbalist. Includes holistic nutrition consulting, education, medicinal herb information, natural health articles, and a health and wellness blog.

Center for Research on Lauric Oils
lauric.org
Provides up-to-date research and interesting links.

The Coconut Diet
coconutdiet.com
Interesting coconut forum hosted by Marianita Shilhavy, CND, and
Brian W. Shilhavy, BA, MA. Discusses coconut and Filipino/Asian
nutrition and foods.

Coconut Recipes
freecoconutrecipes.com
Provides tons of recipes using coconut products.

Coconut Research Center
coconutresearchcenter.org/
Dr. Bruce Fife (director) provides accurate information on the health
benefits of coconut oil.

The ElderCare Forum
eldercare.infopop.cc/6/ubb.x
Advice and support from experienced caregivers.

Nutrition and Physical Degeneration
gutenberg.net.au/ebooks02/0200251h.html
The research of Dr. Weston A. Price.

Oil Pulling Therapy
tiny.cc/eaeahw
Four-part interview with Dr. Bruce Fife.

The Oiling of America
tinyurl.com/6taedow
Scholarly articles by Mary G. Enig, PhD, and Sally Fallon.

Price-Pottenger Nutrition Foundation
ppnf.org
Orthomolecular resources and education related to restoring healthy
function and an optimal nutritional level in the body.

Thai Food and Travel
thaifoodandtravel.com
Coconut recipes and blog posts about the food and culture of
Thailand.

Tropical Traditions
tropicaltraditions.com
Recipes and interesting information on coconut's use and history.

Weston A. Price Foundation
westonaprice.org
Scholarly health and nutrition articles.

References Utilized for This Book

Atkins, Robert C. *Dr. Atkins' Age-Defying Diet.* New York: St. Martin's Paperbacks, 2001.

———. *Dr. Atkins' New Diet Revolution.* New York: Avon Books, 1992.

Balch, Phyllis A. *Prescription for Nutritional Healing.* New York: Avery, 2006.

Baljekar, Mridula, ed. *The Little Book of Indian Recipes.* North Vancouver, BC: Whitecap Books, 1994.

Bowden, Jonny. *The 150 Healthiest Foods on Earth.* Gloucester, MA: Fair Winds, 2007.

Calbom, Cherie. *The Coconut Diet.* New York: Warner Books, 2005.

Castelli, William P. "Concerning the Possibility of a Nut ...." *Archives of Internal Medicine,* July 1992. 152(7): 1371–1372.

Daniel, Kaayla T. *The Whole Soy Story.* Washington, D.C.: New Trends Publishing, 2005.

Dayrit, Conrado S. "Coconut Oil: Atherogenic or Not? (What Therefore Causes Atherosclerosis?)." *Philippine Journal of Cardiology* 31, no. 3 (July 2003): 97-104.

Enig, Mary G. "Coconut: In Support of Good Health in the 21st Century." CoconutOil.com. 1999. http://coconutoil.com/coconut_oil_21st_century/.

———. "In the Land of Oz: The Latest Attack on Coconut Oil." Westonaprice.org. 2009. http://www.westonaprice.org/know-your-fats/land-of-oz-attack-on-coconut-oil.

———. *Know Your Fats: The Complete Primer for Understanding the Nutrition of Fats, Oils and Cholesterol.* Silver Spring, MD: Bethesda Press, 2003.

———. "Lauric Oils as Antimicrobial Agents: Theory of Effect, Scientific Rationale, and Dietary Application as Adjunct Nutritional Support for HIV Infected Individuals." In *Nutrients and Foods in AIDS*, edited by Ronald R. Watson. Boca Raton: CRC Press, 1998.

Enig, Mary G., and Sally Fallon. *The Oiling of America.* westonaprice.org/know-your-fats/the-oiling-of-america, 2000.

Fallon, Sally, and Mary G. Enig. *Nourishing Traditions.* Washington, D.C.: New Trends Publishing, 2001.

Feranil, A. B., et al. "Coconut Oil Is Associated with a Beneficial Lipid Profile in Pre-menopausal Women in the Philippines." *Asia Pacific Journal of Clinical Nutrition* 20, no. 2 (2011): 190-95.

Fife, Bruce. *Oil Pulling Therapy.* Colorado Springs: Piccadilly Books, 2008.

———. *Stop Alzheimer's Now!* Colorado Springs: Piccadilly Books, 2011.

———. *The Coconut Oil Miracle.* New York: Avery, 2004.

German, J. B., and C. J. Dillard. "Saturated Fats: What Dietary Intake?" *American Journal of Clinical Nutrition* 80, no. 3 (September 2004): 550-59.

Graedon, J., and T. Graedon. *The People's Pharmacy Guide to Home and Herbal Remedies.* New York: St. Martin's Press, 1999.

Haas, Elson M., and Buck Levin. *Staying Healthy with Nutrition.* Berkeley, CA: Celestial Arts, 2006.

Holick, Michael F. "Vitamin D and the Prevention of Chronic Disease." Lecture, Symposium, UCSD School of Medicine, 2009. http://www.youtube.com/watch?v=Cq1t9WqOD-0&feature=plcp.

Ingram, Cass. *Nutrition Tests for Better Health.* Buffalo Grove, IL: Knowledge House, 2004.

Intahphuak, S., et al. "Anti-inflammatory, Analgesic, and Antipyretic Activities of Virgin Coconut Oil." *Pharmaceutical Biology* 48, no. 2 (February 2010): 151-57.

Jensen, R. G., et al. "Lipids of Human Breast Milk and Infant Formulas: A Review." *American Journal of Clinical Nutrition* 31, no. 6 (June 1978): 990-1016.

King, B. S., et al. *Food and Agriculture: Consumer Trends and Opportunities: Fats, Oils and Sweets.* Publication no. IP-58. University of Kentucky College of Agriculture, 1999. http://www.ca.uky.edu/agc/pubs/ip/ip58g/ip58g.pdf.

Lavabre, Marcel. *Aromatherapy Workbook.* Rochester, VT: Healing Arts Press, 1990.

Lieberman, S., et al. "A Review of Monolaurin and Lauric Acid: Natural Virucidal and Bactericidal Agents." *Alternative & Complementary Therapies* 12, no. 6 (December 2006): 310-14.

Loomis, Howard F. *Enzymes: The Key to Health.* Madison, WI: 21st Century Nutrition Publishing, 2005.

Mandel, D., et al. "Fat and Energy Contents of Expressed Human Breast Milk in Prolonged Lactation." *Pediatrics* 116, no. 3 (2005): 432-35. doi:10.1542/peds.2005-0313.

Marina, A. M., et al. "Virgin Coconut Oil: Emerging Functional Food Oil." *Trends in Food Science & Technology* 20, no. 10 (2009): 481-87. doi:10.1016/j.tifs.2009.06.003.

Mateljan, George. *The World's Healthiest Foods.* Seattle: George Mateljan Foundation, 2007.

Morris, M., et al. "Dietary Fats and the Risk of Incident Alzheimer Disease." *Archives of Neurology* 60, no. 2 (2003): 194-200.

Nevin, K. G., and T. Rajamohan. "Beneficial Effects of Virgin Coconut Oil on Lipid Parameters and in Vitro LDL Oxidation." *Clinical Biochemistry* 37, no. 9 (2004): 830-35. doi:10.1016

Newport, Mary T. *Alzheimer's Disease: What If There Was a Cure?*, Laguna Beach, CA: Basic Health Publications, 2011.

Nosaka, N., et al. "Effect of Ingestion of Medium-Chain Triacylglycerols on Moderate- and High-Intensity Exercise in Recreational Athletes." *Journal of Nutritional Science and Vitaminology* 55, no. 2 (April 2009): 120-25. doi:10.3177/jnsv.55.120.

O'Brien, John, et al. *Dementia with Lewy Bodies & Parkinson's Disease Dementia.* Boca Raton, FL: Taylor & Francis, 2006.

Ohlgren, Scott, and Joann Tomasulo. *The 28-Day Cleansing Program.* Longmont, CO: Genetic Press, 2006.

Philpott, William H., and Dwight K. Kalita. *Brain Allergies: The Psychonutrient Connection.* New Canaan, CT: Keats Publishing, 1987.

Price, Weston A. *Nutrition and Physical Degeneration, 6th Edition.* La Mesa, CA: The Price-Pottenger Nutrition Foundation, Inc., 1939.

Quillin, Patrick. *Beating Cancer with Nutrition.* Carlsbad, CA: Nutrition Times Press, 2005.

Rabast, U., et al. "Comparative Studies in Obese Subjects Fed Carbohydrate-Restricted and High Carbohydrate 1,000-Calorie Formula Diets." *Annals of Nutrition and Metabolism* 22, no. 5 (1978): 269-77. doi:10.1159/000176222.

Sadeghi, S., et al. "Dietary Lipids Modify the Cytokine Response to Bacterial Lipopolysaccharide in Mice." *Clinical and Experimental Immunology* 96, no. 3 (March 1999): 404-10. doi:10.1046/j.1365-2567.1999.00701.x.

Schindler, Roana, and Gene Schindler. *Hawaii Kai Cookbook.* New York: Hearthside Books, 1970.

Sheasby, Anne, ed. *The Complete Book of 400 Soups.* London: Hermes House, 2010.

Shilhavy, Brian, and Marianita Shilhavy. *Virgin Coconut Oil.* West Bend, WI: Tropical Traditions, Inc., 2005.

Shomon, Mary. *Living Well With Hypothyroidism*. New York: HarperCollins, 2000.

———. *The Thyroid Diet*. New York: HarperCollins, 2004.

Sirinathsinghji, Eva. *Bt Toxin Kills Human Kidney Cells: Cry1Ab Biopesticide Kills Human Cells at Low Doses as Does Roundup Herbicide*. Publication. London: Institute of Science in Society, 2012.

Tholstrup, T., et al. "Fat High in Stearic Acid Favorably Affects Blood Lipids and Factor VII Coagulant Activity in Comparison with Fats High in Palmitic Acid or High in Myristic and Lauric Acids." *American Journal of Clinical Nutrition* 59, no. 2 (February 1994): 371-77.

US Department of Agriculture Handbooks. USDA National Agricultural Library. 2006. http://www.nal.usda.gov/ref/USDApubs/aghandbk.htm.

Venes, Donald, ed. *Tabor's Cyclopedic Medical Dictionary*. Philadelphia: F.A. Davis, 2001.

Index